MW01613570

Joshua's Missing Peace

by

Lori Suthar with Laura Sherman

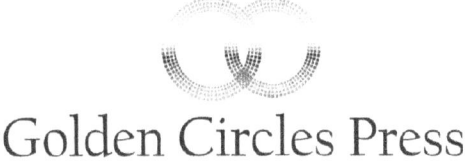

Golden Circles Press

Joshua's Missing Peace

Cover Design by
HolleHock Designs, Inc.
www.hollehock.com

Book Layout and Design by
Jim Kacian
www.redmoonpress.com

Published by
Golden Circles Press
Lori@joshuasmissingpeace.com

For my children,
Joshua, Sydney and Noah
Love you high as the sky and deep as the ocean . . .
And will never ever give up
Promise

Joshua's Missing Peace

This book is intended to share our experiences about our son's medical condition. This book contains general information about a very specific set of medical conditions and their potential treatment options.

However, please be aware that each person's medical condition needs to be individually evaluated separately by a trained medical professional.

The information in this book should not be taken as medical advice. Please do not rely on the information in this book as an alternative to medical advice from a doctor or other health care provider. If you have questions about any medical matter, you should consult your doctor.

If you think you or someone you know is suffering from a medical condition, please seek immediate medical attention. Never delay seeking medical advice, disregard medical advice or discontinue medical treatment because of information contained in this book.

Introduction

When my wife, Lori, discussed the idea of documenting and writing this book, I will admit I wasn't completely on board. I am a reserved person, who believes that our family affairs should be private, not public. Plus I wanted to protect our children, in particular our son, Joshua, from unnecessary scrutiny.

However . . .

Even though I have been a practicing physician for thirteen years, I have learned that there are aspects of medical science that still need to be unraveled. My specialty is the non-surgical treatment of spine related conditions in adults. I generally encourage holistic treatments, incorporating treatments that are lower in risk to my patients.

Although, medications are often the key to many illnesses, we must understand the risk versus benefits of every medication treatment. I am very conservative with medication treatment in my practice. In my heart, I believe this philosophy is even more critical in our children.

I have learned a great deal through other practicing physicians, as well as through research and continual study. I have come to realize that we don't have all the answers. I believe one of the most important attributes to a good physician is knowing one's own strengths and limitations.

It has become clear to me that behavioral disorders are on the rise. We need to research this and discover the sources and causes of this epidemic. Is it connected to the foods we eat? Are there viral or bacterial causes? Are there environmental triggers?

The solution isn't to place our children on anti-depressants, stimulants or other medications that simply mask the symptoms.

When Joshua started having difficulties, Lori and I were new parents. We weren't sure what was "normal" and what wasn't. The last thing I ever wanted to do was put Joshua on any prescription medications. Giving Joshua medications without a clear understanding of what truly afflicted him went against everything I believed, both as a father and a physician.

However, in retrospect, I didn't feel we had any options; Joshua's condition was worsening. We didn't know what else to do but go along with the recommendations of the pediatric specialists.

It isn't easy to expose our most personal family

difficulties in such a public forum. However, my wife and I feel strongly that we must do everything in our power to assist other families who might be facing a similar situation.

May this book be of help to you!

Manish Suthar, M.D.

Hi! My name is Joshua Suthar. I'm 8 years old. My mom asked if she could write a book about my illness and I said yes. I want to help other kids so they aren't given the wrong drugs. Some drugs help and some drugs make things worse. I told my mom to write this book so that no other child ever has to go through what I did.

Love, Joshua Suthar

Chapter One
February 2009

I knew we needed to see a neurologist. There were just too many quirky things going on with our son, Joshua: the head turning, the way he played with his spit, his obsession with numbers . . .

Dr. N had a reputation of being one of the best neurologists in St. Louis. Being an occupational therapist, I had referred a number of patients over to him throughout the years, because I'd heard that he doesn't just slap a label on a child.

Being a physician doesn't always have the perks one might think, but in this case, Manish, my husband, was able to get us an appointment within two weeks. Normally it would have been at least a six-week wait.

I put a lot of stock in Dr. N's opinion. Somehow, I didn't think I was entitled to investigate the warning signs myself, that I needed affirmation from someone else . . . a man in a white coat.

That was a huge mistake.

The morning before the appointment, I found a sitter for my two-year-old daughter, Sydney. I tried in vain to feed Joshua a proper lunch. He just wasn't interested in anything.

Long ago I learned that it wasn't me, I

wasn't a crummy cook. I invested many hours watching cooking shows and many dollars in fancy cookbooks, but the more I tried to be a world-class chef, the farther Joshua pushed the plate away from himself. I liked to blame Manish's non-eating genes.

Growing up in a military family, I was acutely aware of time. We were never late in our family – never. So, I was torn here. Joshua needed to eat a good meal, but the last thing I wanted was to be late to this important doctor's appointment.

My father's training won out in the end. Joshua ate a few bites of a cheese sandwich before we put on our heavy coats and piled into the car.

I smiled as he jumped into his "cow" car seat, a pattern he'd recently picked out. I buckled him in.

"Aw, Mom! I can do it myself," he cried.

"I know, Buddy, but I want to be on time."

"Why are we going to this doctor?"

"Well, he's a different kind of doctor," I tried to explain, as I got into the driver's seat. I wanted to be very honest with him, but not overload him with information. "He's going to ask you a lot of questions and find out how strong you are."

"Will it hurt?" he asked.

"No, I promise it won't. He's not going to give you a shot or anything. OK?"

"OK, Mom," Joshua said.

As we drove down the street I looked at Joshua through the rearview mirror. I hoped he didn't notice how nervous I was. He caught my eye in the mirror and I gave him a brief smile, hoping it was reassuring.

"What kind of questions will he ask?"

"I don't know, but he may have you take a test," I said, sneaking a peak at his expression.

Any worry that Joshua might have had vanished. He's a competitive boy and loves the chance to show off his skills, especially to an adult. "What kind of test?"

"I don't know, Buddy. We'll have to wait and see."

Joshua had more questions for me, but all I could do was assure him that the visit wouldn't hurt and that I honestly didn't know what questions the doctor would ask.

We arrived early, as planned. Manish hadn't arrived yet, so I sat down and waited. I had imagined the waiting room to look like a giant toy store, being that Dr. N was a pediatric doctor. I was surprised to find only two worn children's books and a bunch of average waiting room magazines for the parents. Nothing about this office was child-friendly.

Very few people were in the office. After a few minutes Dr. N poked his head out of his office and motioned for us to come in. My guess is that Dr. N had worked us in during his lunch break.

When we walked into Dr N's office, the furniture was an imposing mahogany. Many intimidating books lined his bookshelves. Dr. N, shorter than the average man, was swallowed up by his large, burgundy office chair.

I looked at the family photographs and could see

that he was a grandfather many times over. Looking at him carefully, he struck me as a grandfatherly type. It wasn't what I had expected, based on his reputation as a no-nonsense pediatric neurologist.

I glanced at the stacks of paper on his desk and was sure that he knew what each piece of paper contained. There was a sense of order to his disorder.

"It's nice to finally meet you," he said.

I felt honored that he knew who I was. He had taken the time to notice my name on the reports of our shared patients. "The feeling is very mutual," I replied.

"Hello?" Manish poked his head through the door.

"Ah, you must be Dr. Suthar?" Dr. N said.

"Manish," my husband said. "You can call me Manish."

"Come on in and have a seat." He indicated a place next to me.

"Thank you," Manish said. "Sorry I'm late."

"You're right on time," Dr. N said. "We're just getting started. Now, Manish, that's a name you don't hear every day. What nationality is that?"

"Asian Indian."

"Interesting! OK, so Joshua, let's see what's going on." He walked over to our son and helped him up onto the medical table. I shivered. This was the day I'd finally find out was what going on with our son, what was causing him to behave so oddly.

He performed a series of tests on Joshua while Manish and I watched. When he was done he asked one of the office staff to take Joshua into a small room with toys to keep him occupied.

My heart was hammering wildly in my chest. Dr. N immediately said, "I don't think he has ADHD."

Manish and I looked at each other and smiled, simultaneously relaxing back into our chairs. That was a big bullet to dodge.

"Which one of you is the perfectionist?" he said with a smile.

Manish meekly raised his hand. "That would be me."

I laughed, feeling more at ease. It was true. Manish had a medical clinic that was as neat as a pin. No germ could survive for a moment in my husband's office. Joshua definitely took after his father in that regard.

Dr. N smiled and continued with his assessment. "Joshua is extremely bright, but then you already knew that."

Manish and I nodded.

"Enter him in every math competition you find, because he'll win."

Manish beamed with pride. "Should we look into gifted programs?"

"Sure," Dr. N said. "You could get some testing done and then see what's available."

"How about homeschooling?" I asked. "I've been considering that for a while."

Dr. N laughed. "Yeah, you can't put a kid like that into a regular public school classroom. He'll fail from sheer boredom!"

"That's what we were thinking," I said with a

smile.

"I can promise you that he'll never struggle academically. If he does, bring him back because something's wrong. You both have a bright child here."

I stood and began to gather up all my things. This had gone much better than I had thought. Then I realized we still hadn't gotten an answer to our main question, the reason we had brought Joshua in.

"But what about the head turning thing?" I asked.

"Oh that," he replied nonchalantly. "That's obsessive behavior. He'll be on medication by the time he's twelve years old."

That was the moment when the world stopped for me.

After hearing about how bright and gifted our son was, I never expected to hear this renowned doctor so casually say that he'd be put on drugs before he hit puberty.

Manish took over. He shook Dr. N's hand and guided me out the door. I stumbled, feeling like the world was crumbling around me. *How could this be happening? I did all the right things as a mom. I know I did. I was a fully trained occupational therapist. Drugging my child was the last thing I ever wanted to do. And why twelve? What happens at twelve?*

Manish put his arm around me. "Let's grab a bite to eat. I haven't had lunch yet."

Joshua was excited. He'd enjoyed all the tests and was pleased that Dr. N had been impressed by his answers. I tried to go along with his happiness. After all, the best neurologist in town had just said my son was incredibly bright and didn't have ADHD.

"He'll be on medication by the time he's twelve years old."

That phrase repeated over and over in my mind as I looked at Joshua's cute dimples. How on earth had we gotten here? And how does having a "quirky" and "bright" son land you an appointment with a neurologist?

Chapter Two

A t least it's not ADHD," Manish whispered, as he guided me toward the hospital cafeteria. The white walls of the hospital had a sickening gray tint.

"That's true," I said. He was trying to comfort me. I tried to let him.

When we arrived in the lunchroom, Manish and I picked up trays and selected prepackaged sandwiches. I held up a blueberry yogurt questioningly to Joshua. He nodded. I guess he was hungry after the interview.

Joshua added an apple juice and chocolate cookie to the tray. When I readily accepted them he asked, "Mom, are you OK?"

I nodded, smiling weakly. "Sure."

It felt as though I was moving through Jello as we walked over to the cashier to pay for lunch. I looked down at the turkey on white bread sandwich and grimaced. How would I swallow this?

Manish took my tray and indicated, with a nod, to a table by the far window. "Why don't you grab us a table?"

I smiled gratefully. The place was nearly empty, as the lunch rush was over. There really was no need to get a table, but Manish, being the considerate husband he is, recognized that I really needed a few minutes to pull myself together. I sat down, glancing over at the boys. They'd gone back to get something else. Looking out the window, I noticed a young woman walking around the courtyard. She was rubbing her slightly extended tummy in a telltale way. I wondered how far along she was. I smiled, remembering how excited I was when I was pregnant with Joshua.

I'd spent the previous ten years taking care of other people's children and was ready to have my own. It was my turn. I stayed up late reading all the baby books, researching the best cribs, the latest toys and all the tidbits of information on any forum that talked about parenthood. I subscribed to a variety of magazines and free services for new parents. I received weekly emails, detailing what Joshua looked like at each stage of his development.

Manish was equally excited. He loved to touch my belly, lovingly whispering to Joshua how much we loved him. We decorated the baby room together, with different shades of blue, sponge-painting blue stars on the ceiling. Later Manish stuck glow-in-the-dark stars all around the room. It was a boy's room.

About a month before I was ready to deliver, Manish opened a private medical practice.

It was a few days before Memorial Day when the contractions started. In those early days, I would type all his dictations for him. I knew that I needed to get his current recordings typed before I went into heavy labor, so at 4:00 a.m. I crept into the home office, timing my contractions as I typed.

Since the contractions were steadily five minutes apart and strong, we decided to go to the hospital. The ultrasound showed that there wasn't enough fluid, so they induced labor.

To say I was nervous was an understatement. I had almost miscarried Joshua the last time I had been in a hospital. The pain had been excruciating. We'd wanted a baby so badly I couldn't bear the thought of losing him. That fear was still there as the Pitocin kicked in and the nightmare of active labor began.

I shivered, remembering how, when I'd called my mom after that ordeal, she had seemed to know. "I had a horrible dream last night, Lori," she'd told me. "It upset me so much I couldn't go back to sleep. I dreamt you were in the hospital crying and I just knew. All I could do was pray."

I knew this was different. I was about to deliver a healthy baby boy, but I couldn't help but be scared. He was three and a half weeks early and I didn't like that the amniotic fluid wasn't right.

The labor was long and very painful. The doctor would come in periodically, check on me and then go deliver a baby nearby. It seemed to go on forever.

Joshua was born exactly at midnight on May 22, 2003. He was 6 lbs 7 oz and a dusky gray color. It was obvious something was wrong.

"Let's go ahead and call the neonatal team in here," our doctor said, keeping her voice calm. We were good friends, so I knew she was concerned.

Or maybe this was all part of having a baby and I was being overly worried.

The team put Joshua on the table and began trying to clear his mouth, so that he could breathe. When Manish and I saw our baby's cone shaped head we both smiled at each other. He leaned over and whispered, "What a head."

As they suctioned out his mouth, I asked what color the fluid was. I knew that this was important, as it could indicate serious problems.

"Tell her it's clear," a nurse whispered.

I was able to hold my beautiful baby boy for a few minutes before they took him away. I tried to calm him, reassure him that everything would be OK.

The neonatologist appeared and left with Manish and Joshua. Our relatives cleared out one by one and soon I was alone in the delivery room with a Coke and a cup of ice.

A few hours later the neonatologist and relatives reappeared. I instantly felt nauseous when I saw the doctor's expression.

"It looks like Joshua had a small hole in his lung. He's currently in the neonatal unit just getting a little bit of oxygen," he said. "The hole will probably close up on its own."

I looked at my brother-in-law with a "That's it?" expression, before shifting my gaze back to the doctor. I waited a few moments before I voiced my question. "Is that all that's wrong?"

"Yes," the doctor said.

I was confused by his demeanor. "There's

nothing else wrong except a small hole in his lung that you feel will close up on its own?"

"That's correct," he said.

We all thanked him as he left the room. It was now three in the morning and I was beyond exhausted. The nurse helped me to a wheelchair, saying cheerfully, "We know you want to see your baby before you go to your room."

"Of course," I murmured. I remember thinking, *honestly, that's the last thing I want to do. I've been in labor all day and I just want to go to sleep.* But I dutifully rode into the neonatal unit to see my son. He looked as exhausted as I was.

After I had slept for a few hours, I got up and found my way to the NICU (Neonatal Intensive-Care Unit), at the other end of the hospital. It was a painstaking process of finding a wheelchair, pushing it a few steps and then sitting back to rest. Finally, a nurse found me and drove me the rest of the way there.

I really wanted to nurse my son more than anything. I had looked forward to it for so long, dreaming of the day when I could hold my son in my arms and feed him. The nurses wouldn't allow it until I had clearance from the neonatologist.

I sat by Joshua's side until the doctor arrived from lunch. He immediately approved my request, but then recommended a five-in-one vaccine for Joshua.

Are you kidding? I thought. I had made it abundantly clear to my pediatrician and obstetrician that we were going to delay his vaccination schedule. After treating children with difficulties for ten years, I seriously wondered about the correlation between vaccinations and autism. I'd seen too much not to be concerned.

I was very uncomfortable with the sheer number of shots being given to babies. It's startling how much the drug companies make every time a shot was "required."

"I don't want any vaccinations for him," I said, "at least not this early."

The doctor looked at me as if I was from a different planet. "Does your pediatrician know about this?" he asked sharply.

I could feel my face turning red. I realized that this would be an ongoing battle. Manish had needed a lot of convincing, too, but when I presented him with enough research to deliver a thesis, supporting the position of never vaccinating, he relented. In the end we agreed to immunize when Joshua was older.

"Yes, as a matter of fact she does. And my OB knows as well, so you can write it on his chart in red pen, NO VACCINES. He's been through enough!" I said.

He shrugged his shoulders and left.

When Joshua was moved to the regular nursery, they allowed me to take him into the room with me. He was just not comfortable in the Isolette (the plastic crib for new babies). He cried when I put him down.

Because he was premature, he was on a feeding schedule every 2 hours, learning to nurse. Needless to say, I hadn't gotten any sleep. Finally, I did the unthinkable and just pulled him in the bed with me. We both slept so soundly, it was heaven.

When I heard the lactation consultant enter the room, I quickly tried to rouse myself, acting like we were just resting. It was no use. She knew. "Oh God," I thought. "They're going to take him away from me."

"Mothers have slept with their babies for years, it's OK," her soft voice reassured me. I smiled a conspiratorial smile and relaxed as she gave me tips on how to feed my son.

Soon we were able to take Joshua home. I imagine we were typical first-time parents. Terribly in love with our baby, everything centered around him. Our car no longer played adult music. It was filled with the sounds of popular children's songs.

When he was four months old I put him in day care at the small school where I worked, but he caught two viruses in the two weeks he was there, so I took him home.

My 80-year-old grandmother then came to stay with us, helping with Joshua until I could end my job commitment. By Christmas I was able to stay home with him full time.

I nursed him for over a year. I don't believe he ever ate any baby food out of a jar, because I made everything homemade.

The kitchen was a disaster twice a month, as I steamed and baked all kinds of vegetables for him, pureeing and freezing them into little ice cube trays. In those days, he'd pretty much eat anything.

Kale and chicken was one of his favorites.

For his first birthday, I made a masterpiece Cookie Monster cake all for him. He loved it, digging into the blue icing so hard it flew around the kitchen like shrapnel. I still find little bits of blue in my kitchen to this day.

By the time he was fifteen months old he could identify all colors, shapes and animals. He picked up on sign language, signing over 150 words by the time he was sixteen months.

His development was right on schedule at every pediatrician appointment. I was nervous and anxious about each doctor visit, but Joshua was always a model baby.

By the time he was two, we learned we were expecting again. This time we were having a girl! I had always wanted a little girl to dress in bows and tutus.

We never sat Joshua down to explain that he'd be a big brother. We just started loading up on pink "girl gear," redecorating the nursery, even though we knew from prior experience that Sydney wouldn't live there for at least six or seven months after the birth. It was just easier to have the kids in our room with us.

I had many Braxton Hicks contractions, which are painless false alarms. One evening, while Joshua and Manish were cooking dinner, I noticed that the contractions were coming close together, so I went out for a drive. This calmed the Braxton Hicks contractions down.

However, this evening was different. Before I

knew it I found myself at the hospital, in heavy labor. I called Manish, who called his father to stay with Joshua.

The next morning, Sydney Lynn Suthar was born. Like Joshua, she was three weeks early, but unlike her brother she was a healthy eight pounds.

We have pictures of Joshua holding her, smiling, that first night home. He was such a loving brother to his "Baby Sydney," his name for her for at least two years.

For many years I'd heard parents complain about their "colicky" babies. I had always assumed these were babies who cried a bit more or perhaps needed a little extra swaddling.

Sydney educated me on colic. I spent many days with her resting against my chest in the bedroom, with the blinds closed. Any noise would startle her, so Manish looked after Joshua. They bonded during those months.

When I took Sydney to the grocery store, she'd be screaming by the time we hit aisle seven. By the time I got to the checkout line, the grocery store employees would run over to help me unload the cart, so that I could depart the store quickly.

I got a lot of interesting advice. Some women would tell me to take my baby home and feed her. Others would cast me disapproving glances, while holding the hand of their perfectly behaved three-year-old child. Sometimes, a kindly grandmother would say something like, "I've been there, Honey. It will pass."

Looking back, this was the point in my life when

I began to not care what others thought of me. I will always attribute this very important skill in my life to Sydney, because, in reality, it was an ability I'd need.

Amazingly, Joshua never resented Sydney. He'd sing to her, read to her and loved to lie next to her on the blanket. There were times when he could calm Sydney better than I could.

In the van, he would often reach across his car seat and hold her hand. He took his role as big brother very seriously. When she threw objects at him, he'd just duck, saying, "Nice hands, baby Sydney!" He was a gentle, sweet, sensitive child. He still is.

Chapter Three

By the time Noah, our third child, arrived, late 2007, Joshua was four and Sydney was almost two. Joshua had become a seasoned older brother. He did a perfect job of keeping his "Baby Sydney" entertained, even when she was temperamental.

Joshua got along better with her than anyone else did. I worried that he always wanted to make everyone happy, becoming frustrated if he couldn't. We did our best to encourage him to not be overly concerned with what others wanted, advising him that it was OK to disagree with people from time to time.

Christmas was my favorite time of year - always has been. That year was particularly magical. The house had been decorated since Thanksgiving, because I knew I'd never be able to get to it after Noah was born. My parents were there too, which made the day perfect.

The children were overjoyed with their presents. Sydney got a new baby doll, which she loved the second she pulled it from the wrapping. She also enjoyed the grocery cart, loaded with plastic food. Joshua got many presents, but the one he was most excited about, the one he'd been begging me to get for months, was the special cartoon video. They were watching it in the background, as they played on an indoor see-saw. I sat nursing Noah, thinking, *life can't get better than this.*

When the children wanted to get off the seesaw, I jumped up to help them, so that Joshua didn't jump off, sending Sydney flying through the air. Joshua did a great job allowing his sister to get off first, but then he did something he'd never done before. He ran over and smelled the seat where Sydney had been sitting.

My mother and I looked at each other with the same horrified look. We shouted a chorus of, "No!" I had trouble finding the words, explaining to Joshua that it just wasn't polite to sniff the seat of other people. The night went on and he just wasn't himself. We all went to bed.

Lying in bed that night, I was troubled by the sniffing incident. It was so off and so unlike Joshua. I began analyzing. The first thing I thought of was that they were all wound up because of the presents. Still, I'd never seen that reaction from excitement.

The only other thing I could think of was that we'd just taken his pacifier away. Prior to this vacation we had allowed him to have it at night, but Manish and I were adamant we needed to break him of this habit.

As an occupational therapist, I had ideas of things that might help with Joshua's new urge to smell things. If you can keep their other senses alive, keep the mouth busy, that can help.

I gave him thick things to drink through a straw, which can work with children seeking to use their mouth to get sensation. We also made very chewy taste treats.

As time wore on, eating became a nightmare. He'd inspect each bite of food, sniffing it, feeling it for temperature, before eating it. If he got distracted, which was pretty much all the time with a two year old sister and a baby brother, he'd just not eat.

I prayed this new development would disappear before he had to go back to school. I thought about many ways to broach the subject with his preschool teacher, Mrs. Belle.

The good thing was that Mrs. Belle had a way of putting me at ease immediately. She was in her late twenties with a runner's body, long brown hair, and a perpetual smile. I always found myself smiling when I talked to her.

I remember the first day I met her. It was an open house of St. Johns, a private Christian school. I liked her so much, I found myself wishing that I could attend her preschool class.

Mrs. Belle's class was structured, but flexible for the needs of the little ones. There was a kitchen play area, many books, a light table with prisms, and a quiet area for listening to tapes and reading. It was idyllic.

Since my mother was in town, I was able to stand in line the next Monday to enroll him in classes. I was out in front of the building at 6:00 a.m. braving the intense cold weather to get Joshua into one of the best preschools in the city.

I found out later that Mrs. Belle had come from Nebraska. The principal had hired her based on her reputation.

I spent the rest of the Christmas break thinking about what I'd say to Mrs. Belle about Joshua's behavior, but every approach sounded awkward. Finally, I thought, a light humorous approach was the best. I recited my plan over and over until we met with her.

I looked her right in the eye and said, "We've had a development over Christmas. Joshua has discovered his sense of smell!"

As hoped, she laughed. "It's probably just a phase," she said.

I grinned and nodded. "My thoughts exactly."

"Children go through a lot of changes at this age. I wouldn't worry about it."

I felt much better after talking with her. I'm not sure what I expected Mrs. Belle to say, but her supportive attitude gave me strength.

It's tough in the winter because the kids can't go out and play. I started Joshua on a listening program, something that is very successful with the children I have worked with. We had Joshua listen to music, which helped in many ways, but the sniffing continued.

It got worse over time. He'd sniff everything in sight. He tried to hide what he was doing by secretively touching an object and then sniffing his hand. I kept thinking that my experience as an occupational therapist should make things easier, but it didn't.

I decided that I would talk to Dr. Trish, our pediatrician, at our annual checkup in May. I put a lot of faith in her. She reminded me of Mrs. Piggle-Wiggle from the famous story book series. She was a small lady who lived in an upside-down house, in a children-filled neighborhood. Parents would come to her and she would provide magical cures for their children's bad habits.

Dr. Trish always had the right thing to say and never sugar-coated things for my benefit. She was firm, but loving, and had four children of her own. I decided that any woman who had four children and a blossoming career had a right to help me decide how to care for my three children.

In February Joshua started coughing, along with Sydney. I had a massive temperature myself, but knew the children needed to go to the doctor. I packed everyone into the car, hauling them to the pediatrician. Manish was working, so I was on my own with three children. Thankfully Noah wasn't sick, but I was concerned that Joshua and Sydney had pneumonia.

The office was packed. Our usual pediatrician, Dr. Trish, wasn't there, so we saw a new lady. She was middle aged with gray hair and a perpetual scowl.

"Have you had your flu shots?" she asked.

"No," I replied. "I'm here because I'm thinking we might need antibiotics."

"This is the flu," she said. Her tone let me know that she disapproved of my decision not to get the flu shot. "Antibiotics don't help with the flu."

I smiled patiently. "Yes, I know that. I'm not particularly concerned about the flu, but I'm worried about a bacterial infection."

She looked Joshua over carefully and said, "He does have an ear infection."

"So it is bacterial," I said.

"The flu isn't bacterial." She was becoming agitated, so I gave up the argument. As long as we got an antibiotic, I was happy. Well as happy as anyone is when their head is pounding with a $102°$ temperature. I just wanted to crawl home and get back into bed.

I put Noah in our monstrous stroller and hiked back down to the parking lot, bracing myself against the freezing winter winds. I desperately wanted to go home, but needed to pick up the antibiotics first, so we fought the cold again as we made our way to the pharmacy.

By the time we got home, I could feel a deep rattling in my chest. Manish took one look at me and went out to get another prescription of antibiotics for me. We made it through the next week.

The next week went much better for Joshua. He was a lot calmer and he quit smelling everything. The odd mannerisms improved and he was eating more. In fact, things calmed down so much I remember thinking, *so this was just a phase.*

I began questioning whether I should even mention the difficulties we'd had to Dr. Trish in May. She'd probably just think I was being neurotic (and quite frankly, I began to think that was a correct assessment).

However, it didn't last. Things started to deteriorate. At our final parent teacher conference, Mrs. Belle recommended that we hold off on kindergarten for a year and keep him in the pre-kindergarten class.

We struggled with the decision, speaking to several friends and family members about our options. Finally, we chose to hold him back, giving him a chance to develop socially. Plus, if he were the eldest in the class, he could take on a leadership role, something that would benefit him.

At first Joshua was devastated, but when he found out he'd get to keep Mrs. Belle, a teacher he'd had for a year now, he decided that he was in fact very lucky. He loved Mrs. Belle. Plus, he'd be in "junior kindergarten" now, instead of preschool. It made him feel a bit better.

The summer flew by. We spent two weeks in Hilton Head Island, South Carolina. In hindsight, all the fresh air and exercise was very beneficial to Joshua. I remember driving over the bridge, looking out at the ocean, just feeling the stress evaporate.

We'd been going to Hilton Head for vacation since I was six years old. I had always associated this location with peace and relaxation. Our condo was rented long term, so we decided to stay at my parents' one-bedroom condo on the beach. We didn't care about the lack of space and the kids thought it was great.

The children spent the days digging in the sand

and playing at the pool. Every day was an exciting adventure for the children, especially Joshua, who thrived in the sun.

.

Chapter Four

By the time school started, Joshua had become more attached to me, so I volunteered to be the room mother for his class. I figured I'd go on all the field trips anyway, because Joshua never wanted to go without me. "One day I'll wish he wanted me around this much," I told myself.

Over the summer Joshua had developed a thing for numbers. My mother gave him a small hacky sack from her recent trip to Ireland. He figured out how to throw it up in the air and catch it, so we encouraged him to see how many times he could do this without dropping the ball.

It kept him busy while the younger two took their afternoon naps. He'd write down the numbers and keep himself entertained for hours. The game lasted the entire summer vacation.

Now, entering junior kindergarten, he could do math problems in his head. One day the preschool class did a counting activity. They were to put a small piece of foil in water, adding beads until the foil sank. Most children would add about fifteen beads before it would sink. When it was Joshua's turn, he got the same result.

He asked Mrs. Belle if he could try again. He

took his foil into a corner of the room, making some adjustments. Then he tried again. It lasted a lot longer and soon the whole class got into the counting game. Finally, Mrs. Belle stopped them when they got over a hundred.

He started talking about negative numbers, too. I asked Mrs. Belle about it, as it seemed like an odd thing for a five year old to learn about in school (and I certainly hadn't mentioned it to him).

"No, we didn't teach him that," she said. "But the other day when Bobby said that five take away seven is two, Joshua corrected him. 'No, it's not. It's negative two.'"

The first few months went well, but when November rolled around we began to see some problems again. The sniffing was back and he'd started playing with his spit, trying to blow bubbles with it.

We tried to chalk it up to another phase, but after seeing him struggle through the Thanksgiving recital, it was hard to ignore Joshua's difficulties. He was so obsessed with blowing spit bubbles that he was unable to sing. It probably didn't help him that the church's pews were filled with people, making him nervous.

Shortly after that, he started turning his head, rapidly, for no reason. I would read to him a lot. He'd sit on my lap, following along with me. Every fifth word he'd jerk his head around, as if someone were behind him. In the beginning I'd reflexively look, too, asking him, "What are you looking at?" He never could answer, but the head turning didn't stop.

I had been introduced to the idea of homeschooling through a local church. I had taught the 3rd and 4th grade homeschool Bible study classes with another instructor off and on for a couple of years now.

As Joshua's conditioned worsened I strongly considered homeschooling him. The idea of curling up on the couch with him, reading, while the other parents slipped around on the icy roads was appealing. However, I worried, was it the right decision?

As the internal war waged, I realized that if I completely screwed up, well, it was just kindergarten. And I would save a year of private tuition. Still, I feared that I would somehow set him back, putting him even further behind.

Manish and I went back and forth on it, but one day Manish returned from a conference, announcing, "We're homeschooling Joshua!"

"What?" I blurted out.

"I met someone who homeschooled their five grandchildren. I think it would be a perfect solution for Joshua," he said.

Wow, that was easy, I thought. *There's our decision.* But as January grew closer, I became more and more nervous. I prayed to God. "Lord, call me spiritually challenged, but please be clear. Send me a sign. This is such a big decision."

Part of the issue for me was that I didn't think homeschooling was right for Sydney. I knew that she would thrive in the school atmosphere, probably becoming class president for all her grades. I'd never heard of homeschoolers picking out only one child to teach at home. Again, I didn't want to make a horrible mistake and I certainly didn't want to appear to be favoring one child over the others.

I got the sign I asked for at a friend's son's birthday party. We were all doing a craft project and I looked up to see a woman I hadn't seen in years. The last time I had seen her, I had treated her daughter. While I worked with the daughter, her mom gave the other children homework to do. Remembering that she was a homeschooler, I quickly slid over to sit with her.

We had a long discussion that day. I learned a lot about homeschooling, deciding it was the right choice for Joshua. When January rolled around, we enrolled Sydney for preschool for the following September, but not Joshua. He'd finish out the year, but then I'd keep him home.

By the time February arrived, Manish and I were worried about all of Joshua's tics. He was so terribly bright, but was having so many social difficulties. We wanted to check with a neurologist, but didn't want to go to one of the many doctors that would stamp an "autistic" label on him.

We settled on Dr. N and made the appointment. I watched as Dr. N muscle tested Joshua, testing each joint to see if there were differences in strengths between the two sides. I knew about this test, because I used it frequently.

Then he took out a little hammer and

checked Joshua's reflexes. Joshua was very patient throughout, showing interest in what the doctor was doing. He dutifully touched his nose and the doctor's fingers, before moving on to the more physical things like jumping with two feet and then hopping on one.

Dr. N then asked Joshua a number of basic questions, like, "Is it morning or afternoon?" and "What day of the week was *yesterday?*" He moved on to several math problems, increasing the level of difficulty quickly, once he saw how advanced Joshua was. He then pulled out cards with words on them, asking Joshua to read them to him. Joshua loved the game of showing off his knowledge and skill.

The evaluation was over rather quickly. I was surprised and anxious to hear the results. I asked him about homeschooling and was pleased that Dr. N agreed with our choice.

Everything was going well, up until that dreaded moment when Dr. N casually laid out the bombshell that our child would need to be drugged by the time he was twelve.

I realized that I had been staring out the window, with my uneaten sandwich still on the tray in front of me. The pregnant woman was gone, leaving the courtyard empty. I looked over to see my family approaching the little table. Joshua was grinning, while Manish sent me a comforting "We'll get through this" look.

Would we? I thought. *How?*

Later that evening Manish and I waited until

the children were asleep before really discussing our options.

"I hate this," I said.

"I know. Me, too."

"It's just not what I planned at all."

Manish stroked my hair as I leaned back into him. I felt so fortunate to have him as my partner in life.

Over the next few weeks I started exploring testing Joshua to find out more about what was happening. Testing is free within the school district, but I wanted to make sure that he wouldn't be labeled in any way (unless it would somehow benefit him).

So, Manish and I decided to explore a private testing center. That way I could control the results, burying them if necessary. I chose a local psychologist, Dr. P for testing. She asked me to drop him off for two hours. I felt uncomfortable with it, but followed her direction. Before I left I gave her a folder of things he'd done. He'd written many books about mermaids, being entranced by Ariel. Plus, I had tons of samples of his math work.

When I came back she advised me that she'd need a couple weeks to review all the results. I wasn't surprised, but was disappointed. I wanted the results immediately.

I sat down with her on a Sunday night. She pulled out Joshua's folder and said, "Now, when he first came in, he chose this toy." She held up a small toy with different colored oils, swirling around in water. "You know what he asked me?"

"No," I replied with a smile. I knew whatever it was had impressed her. She wouldn't open with anything else.

"He actually asked me why the colors don't mix!" she said. "Five year olds never ask that."

She showed me various results. Oddly he tested much better in language than in math.

"May I see the protocol?" I asked. The protocol is the actual test sheet on which Joshua had written his answers.

"Sure," she said, handing it over to me.

I nodded and sighed. "The math problems are vertical."

"Yes," Dr. P replied.

"Well, he's used to either doing them in his head or seeing them horizontally. He's never seen them vertically, so he didn't understand them."

"Well, he got this one right," she said, pointing to a problem of 153 − 36. "It took him a month of Sundays to do, but he got it right in the end."

"He got it right," I explained, "because he did the problem in his head. You probably read it aloud to him, right?"

Her jaw dropped. "Oh, wow," she said.

She mentioned that Joshua had problems with "word finding" (finding the correct words when he wanted to communicate a thought) and that he had obsessive tendencies. She recommended a local speech pathologist for further testing.

She wanted me to bring him in for more testing, but I didn't see the point. Before I left she urged me to visit a psychiatrist, Dr. B. "This guy's the best in the area right now. I recommend that you call him soon and get an evaluation done, in case you get into a crisis."

"Really?" I asked. *A crisis*, I thought. *What would that look like?*

"Yes, his wait list is long and if you need his help, you'll have faster access to him if he's already evaluated Joshua."

Here I came in for educational testing and I was being pushed in the direction of getting a psychiatric evaluation for my son. Clearly she felt medication would be needed, but as a psychologist, she couldn't directly prescribe them. So just like the neurologist, she was recommending I get assistance from a psychiatrist for "yet to be fully revealed" psychiatric problems.

Chapter Five

Fortunately, my mother is a pediatric speech pathologist, so I called her to get her opinion on the "word finding" problems that Joshua was having. She sent me many activities to work on with Joshua over the summer. I also called a local speech therapist, who spent a lot of time on the phone with me, explaining her philosophy. I liked her. I could tell that she was interested in helping children.

Her office was close by. It was plain, but she had a huge toy box, which Joshua loved. I had become an expert at giving my son the speech about how we were going to be visiting someone who would play with him and ask him questions (but not give him any shots).

I did my best to not plague Manish with all the details. He was running a business and I felt that my job as a mother was to fix things. That's the way it was in my family, when I was a kid. Mom just fixed things that went wrong.

Over the summer we worked with Joshua, using our home computer, doing games the speech therapist assigned. I can't say we saw a lot of progress, but he liked the games.

We also continued Joshua's enrollment in a karate program for a short summer session. When we returned from our family vacation, Joshua needed to take his test for his next belt. I was nervous about it. Last year Joshua had tested for a belt and had not received it. I didn't want a repeat of that experience.

Joshua had been in karate when he was four years old and had enjoyed it. It was a very positive experience. He'd achieved his yellow belt, the first advancement.

Last May, right before he turned five, we put him with a neighborhood karate program. They provide a teacher (called a sensei) and use the local elementary school's lunchroom once a week. The tables are moved and voila – instant dojo!

The semester was rough. This was before we knew that Joshua was having any difficulties. During the classes he had some behavioral problems and was given a time out on several occasions. Interestingly enough, Joshua admitted that his behavior wasn't what it should be. He just couldn't sit still and pay attention. The sensei described it to me once as, "It's like Joshua was here, but he wasn't here."

Despite everything, I still thought that Joshua would advance to the next level. It was only when I arrived at the ceremony that I realized there had been a miscommunication and that Joshua would not advance.

I was in shock. I pulled my son outside and did my best to explain the situation, but I could see that he wasn't tracking. He didn't understand what was going to happen.

Joshua was adamant about staying. I kind of agreed with that on principle, but I dreaded the upcoming ceremony. One by one, Joshua watched every single classmate receive their new belt. When it was Joshua's turn, he received a certificate, but no belt.

I had trouble looking directly at him. It was too hard and I didn't want both of us to lose it in front of the other parents. Joshua did an admirable job of holding back his tears. He blinked and swallowed in an effort to control his emotions.

As soon as the ordeal was over I ran to him and hugged him tight. I kept thinking, "He's only five! He's way too young for this."

I quickly grabbed his shoes and made a beeline for the door. When we got into the car I broke down. "We don't have to ever go back if you don't want to," I heard myself say. Joshua just whimpered in the back seat. He was devastated.

At night, he wanted to snuggle, one of our favorite activities. It was one of the few times I could really get close to him. We'd talk about all sorts of things. That night I asked him what he wanted to do about karate.

"I want to go back and get my green belt," he said. His sensei really admired that in him. After all, it is one of the skills that karate offers children, an ability to stick with a course of action and attain one's goals.

By the following February we were hip deep in

doctor visits. I did my best to keep the sensei in the loop with Joshua's developments. After all, the sensei was in a good position to give me feedback on my son's behavior and observe any changes.

One thing that I really appreciated was that the sensei took a special interest in Joshua, but never treated him differently from the other students. Joshua had a lot of respect for him and always wanted to make him happy.

By the time July rolled around, we'd returned from vacation and knew that it was time for Joshua to test for the belt again. Joshua was six now. I asked the sensei if my son was really ready. He gave me a sympathetic "no way" look, but recommended that Joshua take advantage of the opportunity to take the test. He felt that at this stage Joshua would benefit from the experience of testing.

This time I had a chance to prepare Joshua, letting him know that he would probably not receive the green belt with the white stripe that he so desperately wanted. He'd have to hold onto the green belt with the red probation stripe a little longer.

At first he didn't want to go. It was understandable, but Manish and I felt it was a good experience for him to learn about sportsmanship, so we convinced him to go.

The evening of the test was hot and sticky. During the car ride to the auditorium I explained that part of the reason he wasn't eligible for the new belt was because we had taken a two week vacation. I hoped that might soften things, taking some of the burden of the loss off his young shoulders.

I explained that the sensei was being nice by allowing him to test, giving him valuable experience.

Joshua told me that he had done very well at a previous week's practice test, but that parents hadn't been allowed to watch. I suspected his definition of "very well" wasn't the same as his sensei's.

I knew he was nervous, and I started to second guess our decision. It had been a summer session, so there had been fewer classes, making it harder to get the required practice. *Was this the right thing to do?*

Just as we pulled into the parking lot, I heard Joshua clicking his tongue. That was a new one. He'd never clicked like that before.

"Mom, I can't stop clicking!" he said.

I laughed nervously and said jokingly, "You'd better, because that noise will drive me crazy!"

Joshua laughed.

If only I'd known what was about to happen.

The auditorium was huge. We were at a middle school with pull-out wooden bleachers. The parents all took seats on the bleachers, waiting for the students and sensei to arrive.

My heart stopped when I saw my son. He was shrugging his shoulders involuntarily, looking over his shoulders, all while blinking and grimacing. As they began to walk across the floor, Joshua was clearly afraid. He could hardly walk.

Although Joshua had been struggling with tics throughout the past few months, at one time or another, they all seemed to kick in at the same time that day. I was shocked by the effect this was having on my son. All I could do was watch in horror, helpless to do anything. I was sure that every other parent was condemning me for putting my son in this horrible position. They must think that I was a cruel, heartless mother.

The sensei turned to the parents and asked us all to leave the auditorium, so that the students could practice for the award's ceremony. As all the parents were leaving, I ran over to Joshua and knelt before him.

"Let's go, Buddy," I said, trying to keep my voice sounding cheerful and calm. I failed miserably.

Joshua stoically looked straight ahead and said, "I'm staying, Mom."

Filled with guilt for pressuring him to do this test, I repeated my plea, "Joshua, you don't have to do this. Please, let's just go home!"

"I'm not a bad sport. I'm staying," he said, still not looking at me, but focusing on some spot on the far wall.

Over my shoulder I heard the voice of the sensei call out to me, "Mrs. Suthar." I turned, and he gently motioned to the door. Seeing that I couldn't do anything without creating a huge scene, I stood up and walked out the door.

I quickly went to stand in front of the little rectangular window, so that I could keep an eye on him. I knew there were parents behind me, trying to crane around my head to see their children, but I didn't care. I wasn't moving. I saw two other students snicker at Joshua. They scooted away from him. It broke my heart.

Then an older girl, maybe twelve or thirteen years old, came up and sat next to him. She gently put her arm around Joshua, pulling him next to her. He continued to stare straight ahead, valiantly trying to hold himself together.

After a few minutes an assistant came over and covered the window with paper and tape. He explained that they didn't want us to see the routine ahead of time, so it could be a surprise.

I wanted to scream at him that I had had quite enough surprises for the day and I was petrified at the thought of any more.

Instead of throttling the assistant, I chose instead to leave the cool auditorium and walk out into the thick July heat. I just needed to get away, get some space. I was about to lose it and didn't want anyone to see me.

Finding a spot between two cars, I crouched down, sobbing uncontrollably. When I was able to calm down, I called Manish. He had stayed home to watch our two younger children. In between sobs I managed to say, "Joshua's sick. Something's really wrong. He needs help!"

"What's happening?" he asked.

"All his tics are going at the same time. He can't move." I didn't tell him about the other children moving away from him. It was already too much to communicate without losing control completely. I had to try to stay strong for Joshua.

"Calm down," he said quietly. "Tomorrow

I'll make some phone calls. We'll get him help, I promise. Right now you just need to focus on getting him home. Can you pull him out?"

"I tried that," I sobbed. "He won't go. I could pick him up and drag him out, but it would make an even bigger scene."

Manish paused for a moment. "OK, just get him out when you can and bring him home. You need to calm down though. If he sees you crying, he's going to lose it."

"I know, I know," I said. I took some deep breaths of the humid air. I felt horrible inside and out.

I walked into the cool school lobby and went straight to the bathroom, avoiding all eye contact with anyone. I wiped my face with a wet, scratchy paper towel. When I came out, I waited for the auditorium doors to open, looking straight ahead. I could feel the eyes of other parents on me. I ignored them. I was making plans.

I sat in the front row and sought out all the exits. Joshua was only thirty-six pounds. I could easily scoop him up and carry him out if things got bad enough. When my son walked in, I gave him a thumbs up and gestured for him to stay calm.

Each child was required to stand up and perform their favorite karate move. The first child got up and immediately forgot his move. He cried. I'll admit that my selfish response was, *Good! If Joshua messes it up, he won't be the only one.*

It was Joshua's turn. The tics were there, but he made it through his routine. I was really proud

57

of him. He had fought through what no little boy should ever have to confront.

The next step was to get through the belt ceremony. The children who didn't receive their belt were given a certificate. Those were handed out first, before the belts. At least they got something, so they didn't feel left out.

They called name after name, but Joshua's name wasn't called. I was furious. *How could they forget this one small thing?* Now he wouldn't receive a belt or a certificate. It wasn't fair.

Joshua was getting more and more stressed. I did my best to will him to calm down from my seat. They had moved on to handing out the belts. *Hang in there, Buddy*, I thought. *It's almost over.*

I was taken aback when I heard Joshua's name called. We looked at each other in shock. He stood up and accepted a new green belt with a certificate. He kept looking at the belt and certificate and then at me. He then started to stand up to show me, but I quickly motioned for him to remain seated. *Just a few more minutes*, I thought.

The only thing that I could figure was that they had decided to give him the green belt without the probation stripe. It wasn't as good as the green belt with the white stripe, but it was an advancement of sorts. And it made sense. It was actually a brilliant solution.

As soon as they completed the belt ceremony, I whisked Joshua over to the sensei. I wanted his teacher to explain what had happened, so that my son would understand.

"It doesn't have the red stripe anymore," I prompted, hoping that the sensei would fill in the reason why on his own, making it sound like a great achievement.

The sensei said, "I know. They sent me the wrong one."

Joshua tugged on my arm to get my attention. "See mom?" he said, holding up his certificate. "I tried to tell you. It says green belt with a white stripe. I did it!"

My mouth was hanging open as I turned back to face the sensei.

"I don't know what happened tonight, Mrs. Suthar," he said. "But Joshua earned his new belt fair and square!"

When we left the auditorium, all the tics vanished. He had conquered his fears and was on top of the world. Over the next two weeks Joshua slept with the certificate under his pillow.

Chapter Six

Over the next week the clicking increased. By the end of the following week he was always clicking when he was awake. In fact, I could tell when he went to sleep, because the clicking would stop. In the morning, I knew the moment he woke up, because the clicking would return.

He could control it a bit in public, but as soon as he was back in the car, or in our house, he'd start clicking again. Our home was never quiet. The other tics increased as well. Joshua would rub his feet, grimace and blink constantly. It seemed much worse when he'd concentrate on something.

Finally, I called my pediatrician, who referred us back to Dr. N. Knowing Joshua's history Dr. N immediately prescribed him 12.5 milligrams of Zoloft, an anti-anxiety drug.

Zoloft? I thought. *I didn't even know that six year olds could take Zoloft!*

Joshua had never taken a pill up to this point. Before we started down the path of giving our child such a heavy drug, we wanted a second opinion. There had to be another solution.

I called around and found Dr. B, a psychiatrist. He came highly recommended by several friends. He could see us within two weeks, but couldn't take our insurance. We decided to bite the bullet and pay the $700 up front charge for the evaluation.

I buckled Joshua into his cow car seat, kissing his brow. "Now, Joshua, this is a special doctor," I said. "I want you to tell him everything, OK?"

"OK, mom," Joshua said shrugging. "Is he going to give me any shots?"

I shook my head. "No, he'll just ask you a lot of questions."

When we arrived I was pleased to see the waiting room well stocked with age appropriate toys. Dr. B came out to meet us, bringing us back to his office. He had a brown leather couch and a large cushy chair. It looked a bit like a movie set for a psychiatrist's office.

I sat on the couch and Joshua cuddled close to me. Dr. B took some history to start and then asked a number of questions about Joshua's current behavior and interests. Although I had no written report on any of the previous doctors' visits, I was able to give him a summary of those results. Joshua was very quiet for the first thirty minutes, but then he began to click.

Dr. B stopped midsentence, saying, "I see what you're taking about now."

We talked about all of his tics, as well as other behaviors we'd seen at home. I told him about how Joshua needed his food to be just so. Recently, we'd had to reheat his meals three or four times in order to get the temperature just right.

"Eight seconds in the microwave is the magic number," I explained. "He has his own idea of hot."

Dr. B nodded and I told him more about all the different obsessions and tics. "Joshua calls them 'Golden Circles,'" I said.

"Ah, that's interesting," he commented. "Gold is a bright, unavoidable color. And then of course circles are continuous. Joshua obviously feels this is something that he has to continue to do." He seemed satisfied with that conclusion.

I found his analysis to be a bit silly. They were what they were and Joshua's name for them really didn't mean much more than a name. I wanted to get to the root of the matter and avoid any undo sugarcoating.

"Doctor, what are we dealing with here?"

"Joshua suffers from anxiety and obsessive compulsive disorder."

"Does he have autism?"

"Why don't we treat what we know first and give the rest some time. We can determine if there is autism later."

I didn't expect him to say that. I thought he'd say, "No, it's not autism." I started wondering if he was trying to give me little bits of bad news at a time. We spent two hours in the Dr.'s office. In the end Dr. B put him on Zoloft.

The previous doctor, Dr. N, had recommended a dose of 12.5mg of this drug, which I thought was bad enough, but Dr. B wrote a prescription for 50mg. He then warned us that with the severity of Joshua's condition they might need to up it to 200mg.

When I got home I researched this drug and

found that adults usually start with a dose of 25mg. I wondered why Dr. B suggested twice what the average adult would take.

I pray a lot. I like to drive, because it gives me time to think and pray. At night Joshua would kneel beside his bed and pray, asking Jesus to take his golden circles away. I'd pray with him and then also listen next door, as he prayed by himself. Joshua never complained. He never asked why. He just asked for help.

I wasn't the same way. I consider myself a bit "spiritually challenged," so I ask God to show us what to do. I also frequently asked, "Why?" I felt that He always gave me enough information, what I needed to know, but that I still needed His guidance. I never prayed as much as I did during this period with my son. Sometimes I couldn't form the words, but just prayed anyway.

We didn't tell a lot of people what was going on. My friends at Bible Study knew, and we prayed for him every Tuesday morning at 11:30.

Joshua would encourage me, saying, "Just find one more doctor mom. The next doctor might know!" I remember wishing that I had his strength.

Joshua had trouble swallowing pills, so we had to get the liquid version of Zoloft, called Sertraline, so we could mix it with his orange juice. It had a high alcohol content and tasted horrible, causing Joshua to choke and gag on it.

After a few days he refused to drink the concoction and even began refusing to drink orange juice plain, his only form of liquid, so we found the smallest pills we could and began teaching him how to swallow them. We stuck it in pudding, giving him a ton of encouragement.

The following week, a different Joshua emerged.

Chapter Seven

It was a cool, sunny afternoon in October. Joshua had been on the new medication for about a week and the tics had lessened a bit, but he had changed. He was less alert, less bright and . . . less alive.

I had the back, sliding glass door open to get some fresh air. In St. Louis we all have basements, so our decks sit up about fourteen feet off the ground. It's a great place for our kids to play. We had a toddler scooter and the three-wheelers out there. The kids loved to draw all over the deck with colored chalk. I liked the ever-changing artwork our children would create.

The deck had a gate, with a lock, so they couldn't get downstairs on their own. I could see them from the kitchen. The railing was three and a half feet high, so we never had to worry about the children falling over. They all knew not to climb on it.

Sydney and Noah were fast asleep upstairs, so Joshua asked if he could go out on the deck to play. I readily agreed. The sun and fresh air would be good for him. Plus I could get a head start on dinner.

I was humming to myself, enjoying the process

of preparing the dinner, when I suddenly realized that the lovely peace and quiet was a little too quiet. It hit me that something was wrong. I looked outside and couldn't see Joshua. I tried not to panic as I went to the door to look around.

Seeing a movement on the far right side, in the corner, I turned in that direction. I suppressed the urge to scream. I didn't want to startle Joshua, who was laying flat on the four inch wide railing of the deck. His thin frame was nearly camouflaged.

Joshua had never been a daring child. We never had to worry about him climbing things or getting into mischief, as we did with the other two kids. In fact, we hardly ever put up gates for him, because his common sense for danger was always excellent.

But here was my fragile son, lying fourteen feet up from the ground, as if he was in his bed. I noticed that his arms were dangling down, brushing the leaves from the tree below.

Slowly, and very quietly, I crept over to him. I did my best to stay out of his line of vision, until I could get close enough to grab him. He lifted his head and I froze, like a deer caught in a car's headlamps. He turned to face the yard.

I moved as quickly as I could. It took agonizing moments to reach him, but when I did I placed one arm around his back, grabbing his closest shoulder with the other. I stumbled backwards, pulling him onto the deck with me. We both landed on the deck floor.

"What were you doing?" I shouted. I hugged him tightly, catching my breath. "What were you thinking?"

Joshua didn't answer, but looked at me with a confused expression. "Why did you take me off the rail?"

"Joshua," I said. "You could have fallen! You could have been very badly hurt."

"Oh," was all he said. At that moment I knew he had no idea what I was talking about.

Joshua had also begun to hurt his sister. It was like his moral compass was off and he had a new set of rules to live by. He stopped listening to us and didn't seem to understand what behavior was acceptable. I was afraid this new drug had given him a cruel instinct to hurt his "Baby Sydney."

I called Manish, explaining what happened. "We're going to have to start watching Joshua a lot closer," I said.

"What more can we do?" Manish asked. "I mean, we're homeschooling him. How much closer can we watch him?"

"I know. I just don't know what to do."

"Call that doctor back and get him off the new medication," Manish cried. "It's the medicine."

"What, and go back to all the clicking, all the nutty obsessive behavior?" I replied. "No way. Look, the psychiatrist said that sometimes, when you put a child on anti-depressants, it unmasks other disorders, as well. Maybe that's what happens with six-year-old boys."

"What's unmasking?"

"Dr. B said that these drugs decrease the anxiety level, which sometimes allows you to see other disorders more clearly."

"Lori, does any of this sound like our Joshua?" Manish asked.

"No," I answered quietly.

"It doesn't to me either. None of this is normal behavior for Joshua. It's the drugs. I know it."

When I hung up the phone I knew he was right. I just really wanted this "miracle" drug to work, to help our son. I figured it might just need more time to settle into his system. I just didn't know what else to do.

Chapter Eight

The following Saturday morning I was upstairs with Sydney and Noah, picking up their bedrooms. I was taking advantage of a rare quiet moment in the house to sort clothes into seasons and sizes. I never get a chance to do that and was way behind. Manish had gone to play racquetball, so the house was quiet.

With a start, I had that realization again that things were way too quiet. "Joshua!" I yelled from upstairs. My voice sounded unnaturally high-pitched. "Where are you, Buddy?" I asked, forcing myself to calm down. I held my breath, praying for an answer.

He wasn't there.

I tore down the two flights of stairs, heading into the basement, frantically calling his name over and over. I searched the Wii room, a favorite hang-out of his. No luck.

I stopped and remembered a story my mother used to tell me. She had torn her home apart looking for my brother, only to find him asleep in his bed the entire time.

I ran up the two flights again and searched his room. I looked in the closets, in case he was playing a game with me. Panic quickly settled in, as all my worst fears started to tumble into my mind. He wasn't in the house. Horrible images surfaced, as tears threatened to spill. I ran out onto the deck.

"Joshua!" I screamed as loudly as I could over and over. If any of my neighbors were trying to sleep in, I ruined that possibility for them. My chest and throat felt tight and I couldn't catch my breath.

I grabbed the phone as I ran from room to room. I must have looked like a cat, running in circles chasing my tail. Who should I call first, Manish or the police? Should I jump in the car and search the neighborhood? Or was it better to stay home in case he found his way back?

Sydney and Noah were upstairs, so my options were limited. I considered calling 9-1-1, but I decided to look out the front door. I wondered how far I could head out the door and still get phone reception. Of course, as Murphy's Law would have it, I was sporting pajamas with food stains from breakfast and bare feet.

The neighborhood was eerily quiet. The sun was shining and the air was strangely still. I felt like I was on some horror film set. Nothing seemed real.

"Joshua," I cried out from the front porch. Maybe calling from here would help, as if the neighborhood might have missed my screams from the backyard. I figured if I were loud enough, he could hear me wherever he was.

The feeling of despair and panic took over as I burst into tears. I still had the phone clutched in my hand. I was about to dial it when I remembered early that morning Joshua had said something about wanting to play with the neighbors. A short ray of hope surged through me. *Please God*, I prayed. *Please let Joshua be there.*

I ran back into the house and looked up the family's phone number. Panic started welling again. Joshua never went anywhere to play with anyone, ever. It wasn't likely.

After what seemed like ages I found the number and dialed the phone with shaky hands. *Please, please, please*, I chanted to myself.

When my neighbor picked up, I took a deep breath, calming myself. I didn't want to sound like an insane person. However, she didn't give me a chance to speak. "Lori, he's here. It's OK, he's here."

I expelled the air I was holding, feeling tremendous relief. I briefly wondered if she had heard my loud cries earlier. I mean, who could have missed them? It was yet another frustrating reminder that no one outside our home could possibly know what we were going through. No one.

She paused for a moment and said softly, "I'm so sorry. He told me you knew, that he told you where he was. I'm so sorry, Lori."

I mumbled something incoherent into the receiver and she said, "Take it easy. I'll watch him for a while. He's OK."

I thanked her, hung up the phone, buried my head in my hands and whispered a thankful prayer.

I couldn't get these two horrifying incidents

out of my mind. Joshua was no longer able to sit still – he was in constant motion. Sitting in a chair was out of the question. We would do his homeschooling work on the floor.

Over the weekend we were working on Phonics, one of his favorite subjects, when he suddenly began violently moving around the floor. He twisted his arms underneath himself, contorting his body in strange ways.

"What's going on, Joshua?" I cried out.

"I don't know, Mom!" He had no control of his body. All I could do was look on helplessly, feeling sorry for him.

"It'll be OK," I said, trying to comfort him.

"I think it's the medicine," he said, as his arms shot out from his body unnaturally.

I nodded. It was the only thing that made sense. "I'll call the doctor first thing tomorrow morning," I promised.

I called the psychiatrist's office the next day, leaving an urgent message for him to please call me back. Then, we went to a special homeschooling event at the local library. Joshua was completely unable to sit in the chair the whole morning. He wiggled and squirmed, finding ways to "sit" upside-down in the chair. *Pick my battles*, I thought. *Let's see, how many ways are there to sit in a chair?*

It took Dr. B a full day to get back to me. The phone rang in the middle of my Bible study class. I recognized the number immediately and ran out of the room as fast as I could. I stopped somewhere down the next hall and answered, slightly out of breath, "Hello! This is Lori."

"Hi, Lori, this is Dr. B. I heard you called."

"Yes, thank you for calling back," I said. I wanted to admonish him for not calling me on Monday, but I knew that wouldn't get me very far. "We've had some setbacks."

"What happened?"

"I think it's the 'unmasking' of the attention and hyperactivity problems that we discussed earlier."

"What exactly are you seeing?"

His voice was sedate, which I found irritating. "What I'm seeing is that he's acting nuts!"

"I see," Dr. B said. "Can you tell me about his behavior?"

"He's unpredictable and impulsive, unlike anything I've ever seen before," I replied. I told him about finding him on the deck and how he ran away from home.

"How are the tics?"

"They're a little less," I said. "But the attention problems are out of control. Homeschooling isn't working anymore. He was doing so well with phonics and math before, and now I can't get him to concentrate." I gave him the details about watching him flail around the floor.

"I recommend Adderall," he said. "It should settle him down a bit."

"But isn't that a stimulant?"

"Yes."

"But, how does that make sense?" In all my years of working with children, I never agreed with a doctor's decision to pump a child full of stimulants.

"Well, it's the usual medication given in a situation like this."

"I'm sorry, but I can't do that. Absolutely not!" I said. "Joshua is only six years old and weighs 36 pounds. I won't put him on something that will probably decrease his appetite even more."

Dr. B sighed. His voice was a bit strained. "Well, there's a non-stimulant option, but it doesn't have the same effect. It's called Strattera. But I guess since he's not in school now, there's no urgency. You have time, which is good, because it might take as much as six weeks to work."

It was good that we were homeschooling. If Joshua had to attend school like this, for six weeks, it would have been more challenging. I wondered how many parents had to put their children on dangerous stimulants that worked faster, just because they were in school.

"Sure, let's try that." I hung up and went by the office to pick up the samples to get started.

The pills were way too large for Joshua to swallow, so we had to sprinkle them in chocolate pudding. It was a bitter powder, but he'd take it in two pudding cups every night.

Once we started him on the Strattera, I noticed a rash within two days. Joshua was also complaining of a sore throat. I gave him some Zyrtec, thinking it was allergies, but when the rash was still there a few days later, I called Dr. B. I asked him if he thought it was a reaction to Strattera. He said it wasn't possible and that we should contact our pediatrician.

We got an appointment that afternoon. The nurse took one look at him and said, "Oh, that's strep."

Great, I thought, *and I gave him Zyrtec. I'm not exactly mother of the year!*

They ran the test and the nurse was right. We got a prescription for antibiotics. *What else could happen to my little boy?*

We picked up Omnicef, a liquid antibiotic, at the drug store and began giving it to him every day. Over the next few days we saw amazing changes in Joshua. The tics went down and his behavior improved greatly. I assumed that the Zoloft had finally started working and that maybe the Strattera wouldn't take six weeks to work after all. Manish still had his doubts, but remained silent.

Over the next few weeks, things tiptoed back to normal. Joshua was more focused and able to study again. His fine motor skills improved, as well. He was relieved that he could color inside the lines again.

At our next psychiatry appointment, Dr. B seemed pleasantly surprised by Joshua's gains. We told him about the incident with strep (which is actually called Scarlet Fever, because the strep was accompanied by a rash) and let him know that Joshua had had a round of antibiotics.

Dr. B. asked Joshua to rate the "Golden Circles" and Joshua gave them a three out of ten. At the last visit he had given them an eight.

Dr. B encouraged us to continue with the Strattera. Manish and I were uncomfortable with the medication, but the doctor recommended it and Joshua was happy. Life was looking hopeful. There was a lure of normalcy that we couldn't ignore, one that stopped us from taking the medication away.

Chapter Nine

Things continued to go well for another month, but soon after Joshua began sliding away again. To make matters worse, he started waking up in the middle of the night.

Manish and I had a moment alone, not a common occurrence in our house. We cuddled in our raised bed. "You've got to be kidding me! We just got the baby to sleep through the night and now our eldest keeps waking up," I exclaimed.

"I'm beginning to wonder if parents ever get to sleep," Manish said.

"It wouldn't be so bad if he didn't startle me the way he does."

Manish chuckled.

"Yeah well, the bed's high enough as it is," I said crossly. Lack of sleep takes away my sense of humor. "Waking up to see him hovering over me, with the moonlight behind his head is . . . "

"A little freaky, huh?"

"To say the least!"

Joshua came to the door. I wondered if he had overheard us, but his expression told me he hadn't. "Going to bed, Buddy?"

"Mom," he said, his eyes boring into mine. "Can I sleep with you? Please?"

I looked at Manish, who nodded. "Sure, come on in," I said. Maybe that would help him sleep through the night.

Joshua lay over Manish's chest. Manish reached out a hand and gently stroked his son's head. It was a rare father-son moment. "This is the last thing I pray about before I go to bed," Manish whispered. "And the first thing I pray about when I wake up."

I felt the urge to say, "It's all going to be OK. He's going to get better." But I couldn't, because I wasn't sure I believed it anymore.

We all fell asleep early. Manish and I were beyond exhausted. I was in a deep sleep when I was jarred awake by a loud maniacal laughter. Dazed, I looked around and realized that the source of the noise was Joshua. He couldn't stop laughing. I glanced at the clock. 3:00 a.m. Oh, joy!

Manish looked like he was in physical pain. He groaned and put a pillow over his head, but nothing could shelter his ears from the laughter. I lay back against the pillow, just waiting for him to stop. Tears fell from my eyes. It was just so frustrating, knowing it would be another sleepless night for both of us.

Finally, I fell back asleep, only to wake up two hours later to noises in the kitchen. I could make out the sound of the microwave door closing and the beeps of buttons being pressed. My befuddled mind thought it must be Manish preparing an early breakfast. I rolled over and opened my eyes. Manish was sound asleep next to me.

I tore off the covers and raced to the kitchen.

Joshua was standing on a chair with a bowl of something. It was his first time using the microwave. I leaned against the counter and sighed. He was fine.

I looked over at the dishwasher. "Did you get a chance to empty it?"

"Yup," Joshua said. "Did it earlier."

We had learned to run the dishwasher before going to bed, otherwise we'd find the cupboards filled with dirty dishes. Joshua wanted to do things to help the family when he woke up early in the morning.

Often he'd move the clothes from the washer to the dryer or he'd unload the dryer, fold the clothes he found, and put them away. Sometimes he'd mop the kitchen floor. We did, however, draw the line at his using the vacuum. There's no way the other kids could sleep through that racket. There were a few times when I'd wake up and just watch him. He was driven to clean the house. He moved at speeds that topped mine during the day.

I started to develop a 'mommy-radar,' sensing when he had left his room. I'd just wake up. I learned to trust this instinct and managed to keep myself awake, knowing he was on his way.

One night, Manish was on the couch. It was 2:00 a.m., and Joshua came downstairs to get a tin of crayons. He intended to go back upstairs, but wound up at the basement door instead. He had no idea of the danger he was in.

He took one step and missed his footing, falling down the flight of stairs. I flew out of the bedroom at the same time as Manish jumped off the couch. The sound of the tin of crayons crashing down the stairs made my heart leap into my throat. I checked Joshua all over, making sure there weren't any major injuries. He was in tears, but only had a few scrapes from the incident.

After the trauma of the fall, he went to bed, falling asleep quickly. Manish came back to bed and held me.

"Should we call Dr. B tomorrow?" I asked.

He stiffened. "If we call the psychiatrist, you know what he'll say."

"More drugs."

"Exactly. Do you really think he needs another prescription?"

I craned my neck around to look at him. "But he needs to sleep. We need to sleep. What are we going to do?"

"I don't know."

"Manish, I'm exhausted. We need to do something."

"Yes, but more drugs aren't the answer, and that's the only solution the psychiatrist will have."

I turned my head back into his chest and closed my eyes. "We can't leave Joshua alone with Sydney anymore, you know."

Manish was silent for a while. "What happened?"

"It's getting worse. Earlier today, Sydney was just lying on the floor, in the basement, minding her own business, playing. Joshua walked up to her and kicked a soccer ball into her face." I could have gone on about how he sometimes screamed when she looked at him or how he said things like, "I hate you. I wish you were never born!", but I wanted to spare Manish those details.

"How did she handle it?"

"Not well," I answered with a sigh. "I think she's learning to do without a big brother."

Although I was half asleep, and we were discussing such horrible things, it was a relief to have a quiet, uninterrupted conversation.

"The other night, Joshua begged me to not give up on him," I whispered.

"What did you tell him?"

"That I'd always be there for him. No matter what. I didn't tell him, but I was thinking that if he lands in juvenile hall, I would visit him every day. That might be what 'not giving up on him' would mean. Isn't that horrible?"

Manish gave me a hard squeeze. "It won't come to that. I know it won't. We'll work out a solution. In the meantime, just keep an eye on him, and as you said, don't leave him alone with Sydney or Noah."

Because we were homeschooling Joshua, he was able to take an afternoon nap. He needed that extra sleep.

As he progressed in math, the concept of my teaching him became a joke. Math isn't my strong suit, not by a long shot.

One day in the car Joshua decided to quiz me. "Mom, what's four times eighteen?"

I frantically tried to count in my head: *four, eight, and twelve . . . No, that's not going to help.* I glanced over at the side pocket on the door, where my phone was. I briefly considered trying to type the numbers into the calculator, but decided against it. If texting was illegal, most likely rudimentary math was as well.

"Mom," Joshua said from the back seat. "It's easy! What's eighteen plus eighteen?"

Feeling like a bit of an idiot I mumbled, "Thirty-six."

"Good!" Joshua was clearly enjoying the moment. "Now, what's thirty-six plus thirty six?"

I grinned. He was really getting a kick out of teaching me. Before I could answer he chirped, "Seventy-two, Mom. The answer is seventy-two."

"Pretty good, Buddy!" I said.

I had a friend whose son struggled in math. She took him to a local math and reading learning center, where he improved remarkably. I figured that if Joshua's interest lay in math we should encourage it. I mean, that's the whole idea behind homeschooling, right?

I could teach him any other subject, but let someone else guide him in math. It was a perfect balance. I took him in for an initial evaluation. The director, a petite Chinese woman, was gone for some time with Joshua.

When she returned, she smiled. "He loves math."

"Yes," I said, returning her smile.

"We had a hard time getting him to stop working. He wanted to complete the entire booklet."

"That sounds like my Joshua."

We started the next week. Joshua was ecstatic, but after the first week I saw that he wasn't really being challenged. He'd come home, finish his homework and want more.

I realized that this was the perfect solution to his nighttime activities. We requested more packets. Since the learning center had a reading program as well, we asked for two packets of math and two packets of reading every day. This was twice the norm. It kept him busy.

Each took about fifteen minutes to complete, so I made sure to bring home the four packets each day. *That should give us an extra hour of sleep,* I calculated.

The learning center was a place of independent work. Parents sat in the waiting room, while the children worked in the workroom. I would strain and stretch my neck around the doorway to see if he was demonstrating any tics, but I couldn't see him.

One day I caught a notification flyer in his little bag, requesting a parent-teacher meeting. *Ah, here it comes,* I thought. I made the appointment in the evening, so that Manish could take care of the kids.

The teacher welcomed me and pulled out a sheet of math and reading levels. She circled where Joshua was. "He's beginning division now." She sounded impressed.

I looked over the worksheets and asked, "Why don't they do the division down, vertically, instead of across?"

"Well, Mrs. Suthar," she said, "we don't start that until we are dividing with three numbers. That's long division. We're not there yet."

I nodded, feeling foolish. "That's why I don't teach him math at home," I mumbled.

She smiled. "Joshua's doing very well here. We're happy to have him."

So far she hadn't mentioned any tics. I coughed and asked, "Does he make any sounds when he works here?"

"Sounds?" she asked, looking puzzled.

"Yeah, noises or anything like that?"

I could see that she was mentally reviewing his working habits. "No," she said after a moment. "Nothing like that. He does like to talk a lot. Is that what you mean?"

"No," I replied. "At home he has a few small tics. I wondered if you saw them here."

She shook her head. "No."

I felt a little paranoid. *Was she trying to spare my feelings?* I wondered. I wanted to ask more questions, to try to get a more accurate picture, but decided to drop it. I certainly didn't want to create a problem where none existed.

"Mrs. Suthar, are you sure you want to keep taking so many packets home? The work that Joshua is doing now is very advanced."

"Yes," I replied without hesitation. I prayed she wouldn't ask for an explanation.

She didn't.

Chapter Ten

Toward the end of October my parents invited us to spend a week with them in Cancun. I must have been desperate to consider bringing three young children on an international flight. The only reason we could make it work was because my mom was there.

My parents have been married for over fifty years. They are a perfect pair, a constant role model for me. They do what they want to do, when they want to do it. My mother, in particular, is fearless. She said to me once, "I'm almost seventy years old. I've spent my life keeping my mouth shut, worrying about what other people might think of me. I don't care anymore. If someone doesn't like how I am, that's fine. I have plenty of friends who aren't offended by me. I am only accountable to God." At the age of forty, I'm trying to take that advice, and learn from her.

When Joshua was born, my mother was very clear that she wasn't to be called "Grandma." Manish suggested "Nani," which is Indian for "young mother." A visiting friend spoke up, telling her that Nani meant "beautiful" in Hawaiian. My mother fell in love with the name and claimed the title as her own.

When my mother stays with us, Joshua pours his heart out to her, telling her his innermost thoughts. She only tells me things that she feels I really need to know, keeping everything else confidential.

Joshua knows to let her be until 6am. However, the moment the clock strikes 6:00 A.M., he's in her room. She tells me that he often whispers, "Nani, you don't have to talk or keep your eyes open. Just say 'uh-huh' now and then to let me know that you're hearing me, OK?"

She never reacts strongly to what he says, so that he'll feel more comfortable talking to her. Joshua tells me that his Nani is a great listener.

When we arrived in Cancun, Joshua flew into his Nani's arms. Their timeshare was on the eighth floor, overlooking the pool and ocean. Instead of taking in the breathtaking beauty of the view, all I could think was, *He's going to jump off the balcony!*

We spent a lot of time rigging things so that he couldn't get out. He slept with my mom, because she was the lightest sleeper of any of us. There were two doors between him and the balcony, which also gave us extra time.

He was clicking away, while she held him. "I thought he was on medication for this," she whispered to me. "I thought it was helping."

"It will," I said. "It takes time." I wondered if she caught on that I wasn't terribly convinced.

We spent a lot of time in the pool. Mom believes that children should spend most of their day running around outside, getting good and dirty. Manish and I often toyed with the idea of sending Joshua to stay with her for the summer, so that she could work with him one-on-one.

Mom lives in a very rural area, working with children as a speech pathologist. The times that Joshua spends outside, camping or at the beach, he does better. I wish I could find a way to do that for him more.

After the first few days of the pool, Joshua began to get the hang of swimming. He didn't put his face in the water, but he could move his arms and legs and propel himself around. We were thrilled. It was a major milestone.

Other activities didn't go so well. For instance, one day we all went out to paint ceramics. Sydney had a blast, quietly painting her butterfly for half an hour, while Joshua gave his dolphin a few brushstrokes and then proceeded to run around the table for the rest of the time. It was like he was three years old again.

We finished quickly and headed back upstairs. Sydney started to feel ill and later that evening developed a temperature of 102°. I put her to bed, thinking that she just needed a little rest, but the next day she was worse. When her temperature hit 105°, I realized we needed a doctor.

I put her in a stroller and headed downstairs to the front desk. I was directed to the lower level, where there was a small medical office. It was 5:30 in the evening, after hours, so they needed to call the doctor, but they reassured me he'd be there within thirty minutes.

The physician met us there by 6:00 p.m. and Manish joined us in the office.

"How long has she had fever?" the doctor asked in a thick accent.

"Two days," I said. "Is it strep?"

"Yes," he said. "When you leaving Mexico?"

"The day after tomorrow," I replied.

He dug around in his medicine bag and pulled out a huge needle. I grabbed Sydney's head, turning it toward me, so that she wouldn't see it and freak out, the way I was.

I looked at my husband. His eyes were as big as mine. Surely this doctor wasn't considering using this needle on our three-year-old daughter! Maybe he would use it to fill a smaller one.

In the end we had to hold her down while the doctor stuck her in the rear end. *She's going to have a huge puncture wound from that needle,* I thought. She screamed loudly and I felt tears stream down my face.

The doctor gave Manish a prescription for ten days of penicillin. He and my father set out to get it, so that we could keep it in her system. We gave Sydney popsicles to relieve the pain. Within a few hours she looked and felt better.

The next month rolled by, with little change. We settled into our routine and prayed that Joshua would sleep more at night. Soon it was time to pre-pare for Christmas. My parents were coming to spend the holidays, which is always a treat for us.

This year, we decided to celebrate Christmas and then go to Branson together, staying in a time share. It was only four hours away, but was a much needed break from the stress of home.

Joshua was getting himself into trouble on a continual basis. The day after we arrived, in Branson, my mother and I decided to take the kids to a local restaurant. Manish and Dad stayed home to watch football on TV.

As we drove down the street, we passed a fast food place.

"Let's go there," Joshua said, craning his neck around to look back at the restaurant.

I groaned. I can count the number of times on one hand that I've taken my kids for fast food. "Not today," I said firmly.

"No fair!"

"Nani and I want to eat somewhere else."

Joshua wouldn't let it go. He kept whining and complaining. I did my best to ignore him. *Normal, but annoying*, I thought. I can proudly say that I didn't even consider giving in, not for a moment. This was my vacation too!

His whining didn't stop. I could tell that he thought he could change our minds. "Joshua, it's not going to happen. I think you'll like the place we're going. You know we don't do fast food."

"But I want to go."

"Maybe, if you behave nicely, we'll make an exception, and go at the end of the week. Maybe." It was a huge concession, one that I felt was extremely generous. I was sure that would get him to calm down. I was wrong.

"It's not fair!"

"Joshua," I said firmly. "That's the end of the discussion."

"Sydney, don't you want to go to the other place?" Joshua asked.

Sydney agreed that she did. Noah also piped in with his cute two-year-old voice that he wanted to go, too. Sydney and Noah were copying Joshua's whiny demands, which just made me even angrier.

When we pulled into the parking lot of the restaurant, Joshua was in a rage.

"I don't want to go to this stupid place," he screamed. He could see another fast food place across the street. "I want to go there! If you don't let me, I'll run away and go there by myself!"

"If you don't want to eat with the family, you can sit in the car with me and have a peanut butter sandwich when we get home."

"I hate you!" he screamed.

"Mom, why don't you take the other two into the restaurant and I'll stay here with Joshua." Joshua was screaming so loudly, I had to lean in toward her.

She nodded and took Sydney and Noah into the restaurant. I looked at Joshua in the rear view mirror. It was like he was possessed. This had escalated from a "normal" tantrum that kids sometimes have, to a level I had never experienced before.

He unbuckled his seat belt and lunged at me. His fingers became claws as he hit me, pulled my hair, doing whatever damage he could do. I was trying to fend off his attacks, while I climbed into the back seat. I needed to make sure he didn't climb out of the van and run across the street. It is surprising how strong such a little guy can be.

He punched me and screamed, "I hate you!" Then he kicked me and yelled, "You're the worst mom ever! I wish I had a different mom."

"Joshua, I love you. But you are not going to act like this!" I screamed back at him. Sometimes yelling back is the right thing to do. I was glad that the windows were tinted, but wondered what the passersby thought of the screams coming from the van. Hopefully no one was calling the police.

I finally wrestled Joshua back into the back seat and into his car seat. I managed to buckle the seat belt, while fending off blows. I then placed my hand over the latch, so that he couldn't get out. I felt like I'd just had an exhausting workout, physically and emotionally.

When he saw that he was unable to break free he got a strange look in his eye. He started banging on the window, yelling, "Help! Help! Someone help me!"

I held my breath and looked around. What could I do? I thought briefly about turning on the radio, but if I left Joshua's side, he'd unbuckle his seatbelt and it would be harder to restrain him.

Would anyone do anything? I watched people get in and out of their cars, but no one dialed 911. A few shot glances our way, but I guess since we weren't leaving, it was clear I wasn't a kidnapper.

After about an hour, Joshua finally calmed down and we were able to go into the restaurant. Everyone else had eaten, so I ordered something to go and we went back to the timeshare.

After things settled down, Mom suggested that Manish and I do a little after-Christmas shopping, to hit the sales. I knew that she could handle Joshua just fine, so I jumped at the chance to have a date night with my husband.

It felt wonderful going out, walking around, without having a child attached to me. It was dark and we were hungry, so we agreed to stop in for a bite to eat. Not many places were open, but we found a small Mediterranean restaurant.

Manish opened the door for me and whispered, "Let's not talk about the children, OK?"

"Deal!" I was looking forward to a real conversation, one that was about adult topics.

"Remember that place in Dallas?" Manish asked with a grin.

"I was just thinking of the Oasis! That was amazing food, wasn't it?"

"Yeah, nothing like it." Manish looked over the menu, as we sipped our sodas.

When I put the menu down, I became aware of the awkward silence. *Think of something to say!* I commanded myself. *This is your chance for grown-up conversation.* Nothing came to mind. I looked up at Manish and gave him a weak smile. He smiled back.

"It's cold out tonight," I said lamely. *Weather? Is that all I could come up with?* I'd just made things even more awkward, if that were possible.

Manish nodded and looked out the window.

I realized how much our lives revolved around our children at that moment. I honestly couldn't think of anything else to talk about and obviously Manish was having the same problem.

I remember reading that over ninety percent of marriages with special needs children end in divorce. Would that be us? Was this a sign that our marriage wasn't strong enough to survive our son's problems?

We gave up and ate our dinner in silence. After dinner we went to the small outlet mall and walked from store to store. Eventually, we split up, visiting different stores. I went to a children's store and bought toys.

Manish and I met back up again, drove home with little conversation and crawled into separate beds, with one child each, and fell asleep.

Chapter Eleven

When we returned from our trip we started back into our routine. Homeschooling, I came to realize, was a bit of a misnomer. We didn't spend much time at home.

I took Joshua to the science center, Wednesday morning Bible study and the co-op center. We had to cover the core subjects and were required to teach a certain number of hours a week, but at his age we didn't need to keep track of it. I did want to practice, though, as it would eventually be required.

I found that I could teach reading, spelling and phonics. We went to the local, homeschooling co-op for the other subjects like music, Spanish, drama, science and art. Manish stepped in to work on science homework and projects.

The co-op was a great system. Parents volunteered once a semester to help out at the center, while the parents who were trained teachers ran the classes. One of the science teachers had a PhD. The fees were low and based on participation. The teachers were paid accordingly.

The classes had a mix of ages. For example, Joshua's first Spanish class had first through third graders. That appealed to me because I felt Joshua needed older role models.

When things spiraled downward in October we held our breath. I figured the Christmas break might ease things for Joshua a bit, but that clearly didn't help.

One day, in early February, I was dropping Joshua off at the learning center. I was in a hurry, late for my Bible study training. I had been up all night handling Joshua and was exhausted.

I was jogging down the corridor, away from the lunchroom, when I heard someone call out, "Mrs. Suthar!"

I turned around and recognized Tyler's mom. Tyler and Joshua shared several classes at the center. "Yes?" I asked, struggling to keep the frustration of being late out of my voice.

"Hi, how are you?" she asked.

"Good," I replied. "And you?" I hadn't really formed any relationships with the other moms at the center. I just didn't have the emotional energy required. She seemed like a nice lady, though.

"Good," she said. "I wanted to let you know that my son was telling me that Joshua is really having a hard time in class lately." She looked apologetic.

Your son is a behavioral mess in class and no one is equipped to handle it, I translated. I imagine that she had drawn the short stick, winning the honor of getting to confront me on this. For some reason I hadn't seen this coming and I was caught off guard. I couldn't help it, I started crying.

The woman was very gracious. "What can I do to help?"

She was so genuine and kind in her offer to help,

that the tears flowed faster. "I'm sorry. You're right. I know he's been having difficulties," I sobbed.

She nodded and said that she understood. I felt like laughing. *Really, then can you explain it to me?*

Instead I said, "I don't want to bother the teachers with more things to do, but how about if I make a behavior card, which they can check off in class? And then I'll create a reward system for him at home."

I felt like I was negotiating a probationary period for my child. I felt relieved when she agreed to take the card to his class. "I'll talk to the teacher and make sure she understands."

"Thank you." I raced to the car to make a "behavior card." It was below freezing, so I turned on the heater and drove closer to the entrance. I frantically looked around the cluttered car. All I could find was an old ad for a tanning salon, which had been left under the windshield wipers last week. Thankfully, it was blank on the back, so I scratched out five shaky columns on it. I wrote the numbers one through five on the top, marking "Poor" over the number one and "Great" over the five.

On the side I wrote out the classes, so that all the teacher would need to do was mark the appropriate box. It was rather primitive, but workable. I vowed to make a better card next week. I handed the paper to the lady, saying, "I'll make this look much better by next week."

"Great," she said. "I'll take it over right now."

"Wait," I said, taking it back. "Let me add in

something." I scribbled, "1 minute of Wii time for each point earned" across the bottom. "Joshua loves Wii. That will help."

She nodded. "Rewards are always good."

When I got into the car I immediately called the psychiatrist and left a message. "What we're doing isn't working. I think we're getting dangerously close to getting kicked out of the Christian Learning Center!"

Later that evening I went food shopping with Joshua and was just checking out when Dr. B called me back. I turned my personal communication switch to sign language mode with the cashier, becoming one of those irresponsible, cell phone wielding mothers that no one likes.

I did my best to appraise Dr. B of Joshua's behavior, without telling everyone in the store. It was 8:00 P.M. and I didn't want to risk not being able to talk to Dr. B for another twenty-four hours. Maybe there was a solution.

"There's a new drug I'd like to try. It's called Intuniv," he said.

Manish was right. The only solution anyone seemed to have, was more medication. Still I had done some research on the net and agreed that this was one to try. At least it wasn't a stimulant.

As I loaded up the van, I heard Joshua strike up a conversation with the woman in the car next to us. He was reeling off math problems, while she acted overly impressed. It was an awkward moment. I never know what to say. I just wanted to get home, and not have any kind of conversation with a stranger at this moment.

Should I act like I don't know, like it's normal? I wondered if I could play that off convincingly and just leave. Or do I let her know that I'm aware and have things under control? I opted for something in-between. "He loves numbers!" I said with a joviality I didn't feel.

She gave me a look that said she knew a lot more was going on. *Great*, I thought. I looked at my watch, hoping she'd take the hint and let us leave.

She didn't. Instead she started asking Joshua a lot of questions. "How old are you? Where do you go to school?"

I interrupted her, saying, "Joshua is homeschooled." I buckled him into his car seat, feeling like I was probably being borderline rude, but I didn't care.

She nodded slowly, keeping her eyes on him. For some reason I felt obliged to continue. "He's got a few issues, but at the same time he's a pretty smart fellow," I said, smiling at him. "He's doing fourth grade math and second grade reading, so we're not really sure what grade he's in!"

It was important to me that Joshua know I was proud of him and his accomplishments.

"Has anyone ever talked to you about 'high functioning autism?" she asked.

Has anyone talked to you about minding your own business, I thought. I couldn't believe that she would mention this in front of Joshua. I glared at her and got in the car and drove away.

"Mom?" Joshua asked after a moment.

Oh boy, here it comes. "Yes, Buddy?"

"Do I have autism?"

"Honestly, I don't know."

"Am I like Zachary and Jack?"

Zachary and Jack were patients of mine. My kids knew them well, because our families had gotten close. They often came to our family get-togethers.

"Some things are hard for you right now and some things are easy. Some things are hard for me too, you know."

"Like math?"

I grinned. "Yes, exactly! Like math."

He paused for a minute and then asked again, "But do I have autism?"

I sighed and glanced at him in the rear view mirror. "People sometimes like to put a label on things, on people. You're just my Joshua, not 'autistic Joshua' or 'anxious Joshua' or anything else. Believe me, if I felt giving you any of those names would help you in any way, I'd do it, but right now, it doesn't. You're just my Joshua. OK?"

"OK, Mom," he said.

We drove to the pharmacy in silence. I glanced back to see him staring out the window. He was deep in thought. When we arrived at the window the prescription was ready. "That will be $165, Ma'am," the girl said. She was a little too chipper.

"That's just great," I muttered. I wasn't interested in being polite as I handed over two weeks' worth of grocery money for this new drug.

Over the next few days we noticed that Joshua's energy level plummeted. It was a bit like someone had turned down his activity knob a few notches. We noticed the difference, as did his various teachers. Somehow this made me think that we were on the right track. I still dreamed of normalcy.

Life at home was day by day. Joshua would fall asleep each afternoon around 3:00 p.m. I tried keeping him up, hoping that would help his nightly sleeping patterns, but it didn't make a difference.

I made sure the kids went to bed at 7:30 p.m. sharp. We were strict with that. Joshua would lie in bed, but not sleep. He'd drift off around 10:00 p.m. and then wake up again at 2:00 a.m. I was physically numb from lack of sleep and had become used to working at a slower speed.

We rarely went anywhere, but did eat out on occasion. There were days we were so exhausted that the idea of cooking a meal was unbearable. Besides, Joshua wouldn't eat anything but chicken nuggets and strawberries.

Late one night, Manish and I were on the couch. We had finally gotten Joshua to sleep – neither of us felt like moving. "Do you think he's better?" I asked Manish. My eyes were closed, as I leaned against his chest.

"No."

"But he is quieter."

"Yeah, well he's heavily drugged," Manish replied.

"I know." There was a moment of silence. I wondered if Manish had drifted off. "Did I tell you about drama class at the center?"

"No." He was still awake.

"The teacher told me that he wouldn't stop laughing. Apparently he was rolling around the floor. She couldn't get him to participate."

"It's the drugs."

I couldn't think of anything to say. Manish was right.

At our next appointment with Dr. B, I went back and forth on telling him about Joshua's sleeping issues. I had researched the different drugs on the market which would help him sleep and couldn't stomach it. Manish would never go for it either. However, if I didn't get sleep soon, I worried I might lose it.

"How are things going?" Dr. B asked, when we came in.

"Joshua hasn't been bouncing off the walls anymore. He's definitely quieter," I said. I looked over at my son, who was upside-down on the couch. As Dr. B turned to observe him, Joshua moved to observe a few bugs on the window sill.

I finally caved. "It's just that he's not sleeping. None of us are."

"When does he wake up?"

"Anytime between 2:00 a.m. and 4:00 a.m. Joshua always knows the exact minute he wakes up."

"It's anxiety," Dr. B said confidently.

I looked a little puzzled. "Anxiety?"

"Think about it. What do you do when you're worried about something and you wake up in the middle of the night?"

"I roll over and look at the clock."

"Right, because you're anxious."

"Yeah, but I'm an adult and time means something to me. I know that if I'm not sleeping, I'll be dead on my feet the next day."

"Trust me, Joshua's anxious about something." He handed me a new prescription. I glanced over it and was relieved that there was nothing added for sleep.

To my horror though, he had upped the Zoloft from 50mg to 75mg! He ignored my shocked expression. "Since 1mg of Intuniv helped so much, I think he still has room for improvement. His weight's in a good range. Let's put him on 2mg."

"That's a lot, don't you think?"

"He can handle it. The Zoloft should help out with the sleep and the Intuniv will help his behavior to continue to improve."

I nodded and left the office. Looking back, I have no idea why I agreed to giving my six-year-old son so many strong drugs. It is a bit crazy to up a medication because "it is working so well."

Joshua began sleeping in the basement. In fact, he sort of moved in. He sometimes played with his cars in his room, but he seemed to prefer the dark isolation of the basement. It was strange, since my Joshua had always been afraid of the dark.

I encouraged this move, since he was farther away from Sydney and Noah. And he seemed to sleep a bit better. I briefly wondered if not having a clock might help things a bit.

We had three different babysitters during this time period. Kim, a single mom of an adopted son, was clearly born to work with children. She had the perfect balance of being loving but strict.

When the recession hit, she lost her job and became more available to help us watch Joshua. This allowed me to work more. One day, a couple of weeks after we had upped Joshua's medication, she called me.

"Lori, I'm sorry to call you at work."

"Not a problem. Is something wrong?"

"Well, Joshua just sort of came at me."

I closed my eyes and leaned back into my chair. "I'm so sorry," I said. "What did he do?"

"He started by throwing things and then he hit me. I tried to hold him down, but . . . "

"What? What did he do?"

"Well, he bit me."

"I'm coming home," I said. "But first, let me talk to him."

She put Joshua on the phone. He didn't say anything, but I could hear his breathing. "Joshua, is this true? Did you really hit and bite Kim?"

"Yes," his quiet voice replied.

"That's horrible. I am really disappointed in you."

Joshua didn't say anything. I sighed and asked him to put Kim back on the line. "Kim, I'll be home as soon as I can. Again, I'm really sorry."

I raced home, wondering what I was going to do. Joshua did these things to us sometimes, but only to the family, never to an outsider. I couldn't believe that he was hurting the babysitters now.

When I got home Susan, the babysitter with a degree in education, was there. She was a great teacher and could help move Joshua along on his curriculum. I dismissed her and brought Joshua into my bedroom. The drive had calmed me down a bit.

"Can you please tell me what happened?" I asked.

He shrugged his shoulders, looking away from me.

"Joshua, I don't know what to say to you! How on earth can you think it's OK to bite and hit someone? Anyone. Especially Kim!"

"Sorry," he mumbled.

"You don't sound terribly sorry," I said. I was horrified to see no sign of remorse from him.

"I am," he replied. His voice sounded cold.

Liar, I thought. *You're just saying what I want to hear.* I wanted to find a way to reach him, get him to understand how wrong his behavior was. "I talked to Anthony." Anthony is Kim's son. Joshua loves Anthony.

Joshua's eyes turned to mine. "You did?" That got him.

"Yup," I lied. "Anthony is very upset, you know. You hurt his mom." I paused for a moment to let that sink in. "We could go over to Kim's house and you could apologize. You could bring band-aids for her owies."

"And I could say I'm sorry to Anthony, too," he said.

"Yes."

"Can I bring my Nemo band-aids?" He sounded almost excited about the prospect, like he was going on a field trip.

"Sure," I said flatly.

I called Kim to give her a heads-up that we'd be arriving on her doorstep. She graciously agreed to have us over. I let her know that Joshua wanted to apologize to Anthony, too, and she thought that was rather sweet.

When we got to her home, Joshua jumped out of the car. Anthony and Kim came out to the porch. They sat down on a bench.

Joshua sat next to Kim. "I'm sorry, Kim," he said.

"Thank you, Joshua. I appreciate your coming over."

He looked at Anthony and said, "I'm sorry."

Anthony looked him in the eye. "It's not about 'sorry.' You hurt my mom."

Joshua looked a little taken aback. Anthony hadn't accepted his apology. It was clear that he recognized it as insincere. I fought back my tears. Joshua was quiet all the way home. I thought about lecturing him, but decided that he'd probably learned a lesson.

One night, a few months before his seventh birthday, I was snuggling with him in the basement. "What can I do to help you?" I asked him.

"I don't know what's wrong with me."

"I don't know either."

"Maybe that's the problem."

"How do you mean?"

"It's just that these doctors don't seem to know."

I thought about that. Joshua was right. They didn't really know. They just kept giving him drugs to try to handle the symptoms.

"You're not going to give up on me, are you?"

I turned his face, so that I could look him in the eyes. "Never, Buddy. I promise to never give up on you." I hugged him tightly and wondered if there was something I could do to help figure out what was going on with Joshua's body. Maybe there was something the psychiatrist had overlooked.

Chapter Twelve

O ur state is very "homeschool friendly." Every year there is a huge homeschooling convention near St. Louis. People come from all over to attend, because curriculum dealers, toy dealers and speakers are there in droves.

When I reviewed the list of lectures, two caught my eye. One was a talk on alternative methods of treating special needs children and the other was about ADHD children.

Manish stayed home with the children, so that I could go. The conference was packed with people from all walks of life. There are a lot of odd ideas about the homeschooling community being filled with religious fanatics, parents of mentally challenged children or gun-wielding rednecks. Anyone attending this conference would have been disabused of that misconception.

I was overwhelmed by all the vendors. *Stay focused*, I thought. I was glancing through a few readers for Joshua when I realized I only had five minutes to get to the first lecture. I registered quickly, looking over their materials on testing for educational purposes and using something with a metronome. It is an an alternative approach to helping children with various disorders. Using a metronome, it teaches children to complete activities to a regular beat, teaching them to pace themselves. I had read about that before, but I hadn't done any thorough research.

I climbed the stairs, searching for the right room. When I came in I glanced around. The room was only a quarter full. *That's odd*, I thought. *I'd have expected it to be packed.* I chose a seat up front, in the center, so I wouldn't miss anything.

The speaker came in and started talking about family dynamics and his daughter with special needs. *I'm in the wrong room*, I panicked. I looked around and groaned. There was no way to leave inconspicuously.

I had two choices. Sit there and miss the lecture I desperately wanted to hear or get up and probably make the speaker feel badly. I thought for a moment and then started to cough a little. I looked at the speaker apologetically and then began coughing "uncontrollably."

I tucked my head down, patting my chest as I did a great rendition of spasmodic coughing and slipped out of the room. *Good, no one will think ill of the speaker. Just me.*

I looked over the program again and found the correct room. Of course the lecture had started, and the room was completely full, but people were standing in the back, so I joined them. I could see the screen in the front of the room. The speaker was excellent. His research was very thorough and fascinating.

The doctor was engrossed in a discussion of

neurology and what happens with children of various disorders. In school I was completely bored by anatomy, but neurology always interested me. Parents asked various questions about alternative treatments to drugs for children with ADHD and other difficulties.

After the lecture I entered a drawing for some kind of evaluation. It included a special study with goggles to test eye movement. I entered it thinking, *Yeah, right. I never win anything. Why on Earth am I entering?*

Two weeks later I received a call from the doctor's office. I had won the drawing! I was very excited (and a little shocked). We set the date for the evaluation.

I told Joshua about the visit. "OK, but will it hurt?"

"No, Buddy."

"What's going to be different with this one?"

Good question, I thought. "Well for one thing they're going to do some cool tests with goggles!"

That was the right thing to say. He was super excited. "Oh, boy!"

"Yeah, it should be fun."

"Why didn't we do this before?"

"Well, I actually won this visit with the doctor!" I said.

"Really? It's free?"

"Yeah!"

"Maybe this is the doctor that will really help me."

I remembered Joshua's words from almost

exactly a year ago, *"Just find one more doctor, Mom. The next doctor might know!"* This could very well be the doctor who knew what was wrong!

When we arrived at the office we were immediately taken to the consultation room. Dr. C entered soon after and asked several questions, giving Joshua a basic neurological exam.

Next he put special goggles on him, which had little cameras built in that could track eye movement. Even small motion could be detected.

Having recently learned about these tests at a conference, Joshua's results shocked me. His eye movement was extremely jittery. He had difficulty tracking objects and seemed to have trouble focusing on a target.

Another doctor came in, which gave me another clue that Joshua's results weren't normal. The two men seemed very interested in Joshua's test. Finally Dr. C said that he would write up a report and then we could sit down and discuss the results in about two weeks.

Two weeks later we met and he recommended the Interactive Metronome Therapy and a neurofeedback treatment that I'd read about at the conference. Neurofeedback is like a video game hooked up to the child's brain. He gave me information to take home to Manish as well.

I was having difficulty reading the neurological report. What I really needed was an unbiased opinion. It took me a while to remember that Lesley, my boss, was married to a neurologist, who specializes in sleep disorders. Maybe he'd look at the report for me.

Lesley was the mother hen of our office. If you need help, she's there for you. I poked my head into her office the next day. "Hi!"

"What can I do for you, doll?"

"Joshua received an eval from a chiropractic neurologist," I began. When Lesley raised an eyebrow I laughed. "Yeah, I don't exactly know what that means either, but he really seems to know his stuff."

She nodded. "How did it go?"

"Well, I saw some scary stuff when they tested Joshua. He wasn't able to track much of anything. I was right there in the room watching." I described the test in detail.

"How can I help?"

"Well, I thought maybe Dan could take a look at the report. And maybe tell me what he thinks?"

She took the evaluation. "And make sure this doctor isn't a quack?"

I smiled. "Something like that."

"I'll give it to him," he promised.

"Thank you so much!" I said, and ran out the door to go back to work.

A few days later I was busy getting the kids to bed. The phone rang and I picked up, as I sorted through Sydney's PJs. *Which one is clean enough for her to wear tonight?*

"Hello?"

"Is this Lori?"

"Yes, this is she." The pink butterfly pajamas would have to do. I was trying to will Sydney to come closer to me, so that I could put the PJs on her while I talked on the phone.

"This is Dan."

Dan? Who's Dan? I thought. *Darn, I wish I had bothered to check the caller ID before I picked up.* Then it clicked. *Dan, Manish's friend!* "Oh, hello! You want to talk to Manish, right?"

"No," he said. "Lesley gave me this evaluation to read . . . "

"Oh, right! Sorry!" I dropped the PJs and put my full attention on the call. "Thank you so much for calling me back. And so quickly! What did you think of the report?"

He asked me a few questions about Joshua and I gave him a brief history. I told him about Dr. B and how we had put him on high doses of Zoloft to handle the tics.

"Really? I'm surprised," he said.

"Why?"

"Well, without getting too technical, Zoloft wouldn't handle tics. I mean it could do something, but not on the level you're talking about."

"But they went away quickly with the stuff," I said.

"Has he ever had any type of infection? I mean around the time this all started?"

All the neurological talk and now discovering that Zoloft didn't actually handle the tics was making me dizzy. "No, not that I know of."

"It's just that I've been reading about this thing called PANDAS. OCD, Tourette's, ADHD and all the other disorders like these can sometimes be linked to infection."

"Right, I'll look into that," I said. I was stuck on the fact that the Zoloft we'd been cramming down Joshua's throat wasn't actually what had handled the tics. I thanked him for calling and hung up the phone.

We were going on vacation in a few weeks. I desperately needed some time away with Manish, time to think and space to actually get some sleep and sort things out.

Chapter Thirteen

Time slipped by and Joshua's seventh birthday was fast approaching. We'd missed Sydney's birthday last January, so I figured we'd combine the two parties and hold it at the local pizza and game place.

I was pleased that I had given myself a week to plan. I had just received an electronic invitation (e-vite) from a family for a birthday party, so I wanted to give that a chance. It seemed like a fun and easy way to send out invitations. I plugged in the names and e-mail addresses of the children's friends and hit send.

Next, I ordered two special cakes for them. They might be able to share a party, but they each needed a separate cake. Joshua was really into soccer, so I got him a beautiful soccer ball cake and Sydney got a lovely butterfly one. I then reserved the Friday afternoon at the pizza place and patted myself on the back for a job well done.

As the week rolled by I didn't notice that no one had replied to the invitations. I was backing out of the driveway Friday morning, on my way to work, when it suddenly hit me that no one had RSVP'd. My heart sank when I realized that no one was coming to the party. I stopped the car and ran over to my neighbor's house. I rang the doorbell a few times.

Karen answered the door. "Hi, Lori!" She looked at me and immediately became worried. "Is everything OK? Joshua, Sydney, Noah?"

"Yes, thank you," I said, realizing that I must be showing my panic on my face. "It's just that I didn't hear back from you about the birthday party tonight and I wanted to make sure you got the invitation."

Karen shook her head. "No, sorry!"

I tried to put on a bright face. "Well, we're going to have a fun time at the pizza party place. Pizza and cake. Do you think you can make it?" I felt myself holding my breath.

"I'm so sorry, Lori," Karen replied. "I just had no idea. I'll see what I can do though. If we can make it, we will, OK?"

"That's all I can ask," I said. "Thank you. And please, you don't need to bring a gift. It would just be amazing if you came. It looks like my e-vites didn't make it out."

I got back into my car. As I pulled out of the driveway I called Manish. He comforted me, telling me it would all work out. He also reminded me that his family would be there.

I tried to sound reassured as I said good-bye, but there was no way that having a bunch of adults would make up for having no one from Joshua's friend list there. I started texting everyone I had invited, or thought I'd invited. I started thinking about the worst-case scenario. As I drove to work

I realized that Sydney would be fine with whatever happened. After all, she was only four. She'd be OK as long as we had the butterfly cake.

However, this could potentially be a disaster for Joshua. After everything that he was going through, this could scar him. I started picturing Joshua sitting at the long table with all the place settings set up, pizzas waiting to be eaten, but no friends. That wasn't going to happen.

During my break I called my friend Beth. She and her daughter had been in my Bible study group. She had four kids, one of whom played soccer with Joshua. Wouldn't it be great if she could come?

I got her voicemail. Darn! I tried to sound calm. "Hey Beth, if you don't want to cook tonight, bring the family to have pizza for Joshua's birthday. I know this is last-minute notice but my e-cards did not work and I didn't realize it until this morning. Don't bring a gift, just bring your kids." OK, that wasn't too bad.

I called a few of Sydney's friends, getting two confirms. Whew! Now I just had to make sure Joshua had friends there, too.

The day went by excruciatingly slowly. I had trouble focusing on work. All I wanted to do was go door-to-door to all of Joshua's schoolmates, trying to interest them in free pizza and cake.

I left work early to pick up the cakes. On the way, the cell phone rang. It was Beth.

I answered the phone, "Beth! Did you get my message? Can you come?"

"Yes, I'll be there."

"All of you?" I asked hopefully.

She laughed. "Yes. All of us!"

"Oh, Beth!" I cried tearfully. "You don't know what this means to me. To us. To Joshua. Thank you so much!"

"I know what you've been through this year, and I know how important Joshua's birthday party is."

"Yes, it is. I've been stressing all day."

"I could hear it in your voice," she said. "That's why I called John's mom. You know John, right?"

"Yeah, I think so."

"He's in some of Joshua's classes. Anyway, they would like to come, too. Plus John has a younger sister. I think Sydney would love her. I mean, I hope it was OK that I invited people to your party, but you sounded so upset . . . "

"Beth, that's perfect! You're a life saver!! Thank you!"

"Don't mention it."

"Do you think I should call her?"

"No, you have enough on your mind. I'll confirm her. See you tonight!"

I hung up the phone and was greatly relieved. Joshua wouldn't be sitting at that long table all by himself. It felt like a great weight had been lifted off my shoulders. I almost skipped as I picked up the cakes.

When we got home, Manish and I quickly got all the kids ready. Joshua was really excited. I realized that I needed to prep him for a small crowd. I tried to explain about the e-vites, but he wasn't listening.

We were the first ones to arrive. There were ten place settings, the minimum required. *OK, so we won't fill the table, but at least they'll both have a couple of friends at their party.*

As we sat down, I looked up to see my neighbor Karen's huge smile. She and her four kids had arrived. I was so excited I jumped up and rushed over to her.

"Hi! I'm so glad you came. Thank you!" I said, barreling into her arms.

"I wouldn't have missed it for the world," she replied.

Beth and her family showed up soon after, as did John and his family. Then my co-teacher from Bible study walked in with her four-year-old daughter. People kept trickling in. I felt giddy, as I kept asking the helper at the pizza place for new place settings. In the end we had nineteen guests, not including our family.

"Joshua looks so happy," Manish said to me, wrapping his arm around me, as I watched the children shooting basketballs into the hoops. Joshua was fighting the tics, but was beside himself with joy. Sydney was nearby, enjoying another game with John's sister.

"He does, doesn't he? Sydney, too."

"You did good, Mama!"

"Thank you," I said, blushing. *I did, didn't I?* "Really, our friends came through for us. I'll never take my friendships for granted again."

Later, the large group sang a raucous "Happy Birthday," which left me in tears. The look of utter wonder on the faces of my children is something I will not soon forget.

Chapter Fourteen

M anish and I vowed to always take a vacation together, alone, once a year. We take a break from parenting, rekindling our relationship, giving ourselves a chance to "date" again. It's like going back to a time when we had no need for a schedule, no children sleeping between us in our bed each night, and no need to prepare meals for five hungry, finicky people. I believe that this agreement is one of the reasons why our marriage has weathered the storms of the last few years.

The first time we left Joshua alone with my parents I was a bit of a wreck. I worried about every little thing and changed my mind about going away a dozen times. I collected thermometers, medicines, insurance cards, social security cards and anything else I thought my parents might need for the two weeks we were gone.

I remember the first few days being miserable. I missed Joshua like mad. However, by the end of the trip, we were both certain that we needed to do this each and every year (maybe more).

This year was tough and I found myself having second thoughts. Still I knew my parents could handle anything that came up. My mom could tame a Tasmanian devil.

Mom assured me that he wouldn't have time to

act up. She's a planner and was well aware of what was happening with him. They had two weeks of outdoor adventure, complete with camping and water parks, scheduled. Mom also knew that I needed a break.

This year Manish and I decided on a cruise around the Bahamas, which included a stop at Key West. I love key lime pie. I joked with Manish that my whole goal for the cruise was to have a margarita and a slice of key lime pie. We both agreed that we needed sleep and a chance to just rest and breathe together.

My parents gave me an e-reader as an early birthday present. It was perfect. I could catch up on my reading during the trip. I allowed myself one "Joshua book," but swore that the rest must be frivolous fun books, ones I'd never have a chance to read at home.

I typed "OCD" into the reader and found a book about a boy who "caught" OCD, called, "Saving Sammy." I bought it immediately, promising myself that if it didn't have enough information, I'd allow myself to pick another Joshua book. Looking back on it, I see how pathetic I was, trying to cheat myself into an extra book for my obsession.

I picked out another few books before we boarded the ship. The first night onboard I started with a great mystery novel. It was so enjoyable that I ignored Manish next to me, finishing it at 2:00 a.m.

The next morning I slept in, a luxury that had become foreign to me. I woke up at 10:00 a.m.

when Manish snuck in after breakfast. I felt like a new woman.

Manish and I spent the first two days in the cabin, reading, watching movies, cuddling and sleeping. We turned into vegetables, very happy vegetables. Normally on a cruise we'd go on as many excursions as we could, staying out of our room. This time we agreed not to plan to do much of anything.

We don't normally watch TV on cruises, but this time we both relished the complete luxury of mindless entertainment. They had old reruns of "I Love Lucy." We watched dozens of shows, laughing together at the silliness.

On the third day we landed in Key West. We walked around the town, holding hands. We were both a bit dazed by the insane amount of sleep we'd had over the last two days.

It was hot, but I didn't mind. I felt completely connected with Manish again, like we did when we were honeymooning. He took pictures all day and we strolled around, holding hands. I had my best friend back again. We bought a few trinkets for the kids, but other than that we had no desire to talk about them. This was our time.

By the end of the day, I felt very refreshed. I decided to start reading "Saving Sammy," a story about a boy with similar symptoms to Joshua. At first I was a little disappointed that it was just a story, but as I got into it I realized that there were strong parallels.

The next day was a reading day. We were on

our way to Nassau and there wasn't much to do. Neither Manish nor I enjoy sunbathing, so we stayed in the cabin. I continued to read "Saving Sammy."

Sammy's symptoms were a bit more severe, but I was stunned to learn that it was all due to an infection. I remembered walking into the pediatrician's office, where the nurse said, "Oh that's strep!" A flood of memories hit me and I realized that he immediately got better after taking the antibiotic. Dan had asked about infections. Could this be similar? *No way. This is just a story*, I thought.

I continued reading and couldn't shake the feeling that this was very important. I didn't put the book down until I finished. I looked over at Manish, who was sleeping peacefully, with his book on his chest.

"Manish?" I asked quietly, hoping that he might wake up.

"Hmm?"

"This book was fascinating."

"The Joshua book?"

"Yeah."

His eyes were still closed. "What did it say?"

"The boy had a strep infection. It's called PANDAS."

"Like the bear?"

"Sort of," I said with a grin. I flipped back through the book. "It stands for Pediatric Autoimmune Neuropsychiatric Disorders Associated with Streptococcal infections."

"That's a mouthful. So, how does this constitute a Joshua book then?"

"Well, that's the thing. Sammy had a lot of the same symptoms as Joshua, just a bit more pronounced."

"Really? And it was a strep infection?" His eyes were open by now.

"That's what this book says. You know, Dan said to check out PANDAS, too."

Manish thought for a while. "Dan knows his stuff. What happened with Sammy? I take it there's a happy ending since the title is "Saving Sammy.""

"Yeah, his mom figured it out. He needed antibiotics. He's doing well."

"And he was psychotic before?"

I nodded. "Pretty much."

"Wow!"

"Yeah, I mean Joshua did have strep right after we put him on all the medication. What if he got better because of the antibiotic, not the Zoloft?" Manish thought for a moment. "Didn't Dan say that the Zoloft wouldn't have made those changes?"

"Yeah, I know. I can't get that out of my mind."

"We should check into it."

"The only thing is that it's a bit controversial."

"I'd be surprised if it wasn't."

I looked up at Manish. "Why?"

"If an antibiotic can cure psychotic behavior in kids, there goes a huge chunk of change for the psychiatric profession."

I nodded. "But do you think Joshua has PANDAS?"

Manish shrugged. "It's possible."

"You don't think he does, do you?"

He looked at me. "I just don't want to see you get your hopes up. I mean the chances are one in a million, right?"

"Maybe, but I'd like to get him tested."

"Definitely, I agree. It can't hurt!"

Since we couldn't do anything until we returned, we continued to devote the rest of the vacation to our relationship. We enjoyed the Bahamas and bought a few more gifts for friends back home. I picked up a few T-shirts and Manish took more pictures.

We visited Atlantis and enjoyed just sitting in front of the aquarium for half an hour. Manish put his arm around me, as we watched fish peacefully swimming around without a care in the world. It was mesmerizing.

The last evening we stayed up late, enjoying a hilarious comedy show. It had been a long time since we'd laughed that hard.

The next day we picked Noah up from my parents. We thought it would be fun to spend a little one-on-one time with him, allowing Joshua and Sydney more time with their grandparents. I briefly considered scrapping that plan and getting Joshua tested for strep, but didn't want to interrupt their plans. Joshua was looking forward to a week at the beach with them.

A week later we met my parents halfway, at a restaurant in Tennessee, to pick up Joshua and Sydney. While we waited for the food my father took the kids outside to give Mom and me a chance to catch up.

When they were out of sight I said, "OK, Mom, tell me the truth. How was he, on a scale of one to ten? One being so bad that you wanted to send him home and ten's a perfect angel."

"The first week he was about a two," she said.

I grinned, looking at her, expecting her to laugh back. She didn't. My smile vanished. "No joke?"

"You have a problem," she said.

"What happened?" I asked with a gulp.

"Well, when we took them to a water park one day, Joshua and Sydney were waiting on the stairs. Suddenly Joshua just pushed Sydney down the stairs of a waterslide."

"What?" I cried. I looked around to make sure no one was looking. I lowered my voice. "Why did he do that?"

"I asked him," she said quietly, "and he said, 'I didn't like the way she was standing.'"

I closed my eyes. It was getting worse, not better. I could hear Joshua's coldness, through my mother's voice. "What did you do?"

"Took him back to the camper and took everything I could think of away from him. No ice cream, no toys, no fun."

"Was Sydney OK?"

"Not really," she said sadly. "She was limping around for several days after."

I looked out the window at my daughter and saw that she was running around playing. "She looks to be pretty well recovered now."

"Yes, she's fine now."

"I'm surprised you agreed to take him a second week. Why didn't you tell me about this when we met in Florida last week to pick up Noah?"

Mom paused for a moment. "Because things were getting better. Being outdoors all that time was starting to have a good effect. The rest of the week went better. And the second week was actually fun. He did a lot of inner tubing and swimming."

"Still, you should have told me."

"I didn't want to worry you," she said.

I nodded. "Listen, I wanted to tell you that I plan to wean him off the psych medicines."

"I think that's a great idea!" she said with a smile. "I never liked the idea of his being on those drugs. They're dangerous."

"I think you're right," I said. "On the cruise I read a book about this boy who was acting like Joshua, but worse. It turned out he had something called PANDAS. Long story short, it's very treatable, and with antibiotics, not antipsychotics."

"You need to get him tested immediately!" she said.

"I know. It's still a long shot, but—"

She cut me off. "It doesn't matter. Besides, I have a good feeling about this."

"Either way, I'm realizing I need to take him off those drugs."

The food came and Dad came back with the kids, so we stopped talking about Joshua and PANDAS. I looked over at my mom. She looked relieved and I felt a bit better.

When we got home, Joshua had another outburst of anger. He was violent and crazy. The next day we called the pediatrician. As luck had it, Mindy, the nurse I knew well was on the phone. She'd known Joshua since he was a baby.

"I'm so glad you picked up. I need your help! We'd like to order an ASO titer for Joshua. Can you do that?" I held my breath. An ASO titer gives you the level of strep antibodies in the blood, which tells you if the person has had strep in the last three to six weeks.

Mindy hesitated. Her cheerful voice dampened slightly. "I'll ask, but . . . "

"But what?"

"It's extremely controversial. I know what you're looking at here and I just don't know."

What's the big deal? I thought. "Well, please give Dr. Trish the message and let me know, OK?"

She agreed. I hung up and called Manish. "I don't think she's going to run the test," I blurted out.

"Why not?" he asked. "It's just a blood test."

"Well, someone's going to call me to let me know. Mindy said it's controversial."

"Wait for Dr. Trish to call you back. I'm not a pediatrician, but it shouldn't be a problem."

I put the cell ringer on high and went on with my day. The next day at work, I got a call. It was Dr. Trish herself.

"I heard you called about an ASO titer for Joshua," she said. Her voice was chipper, a good sign.

"Yes," I replied. I briefed her on the research I'd done and shared my concerns about the psych drugs. "I just don't think it was the Zoloft that made things better. In fact, I think it may be making things worse."

"What do you think it was then?"

"The antibiotics."

"Yeah, I've heard of that theory. PANDAS, right? I don't know if I agree with it, but I'm also not ready to say there's nothing to it. There's not a lot out on PANDAS and the only treatments are antibiotics or IVIG."

"IVIG? What's that?"

"Intravenous immunoglobulin. It's a blood product, administered intravenously."

"I don't think we're going there. From what I understand, antibiotics should do the trick."

"I don't have a problem ordering the test. I just want to know what you're going to do with the numbers."

The truth was that I had no clue what I was going to do with the numbers. If they came back high, we'd figure it out. "Can we just try him on a round of antibiotics and see what happens?"

I held my breath. Dr. Trish was very cautious about antibiotics. They aren't harmless. *That was a stupid request*, I thought. *I probably just blew it.*

I was surprised when she came back with a quick answer. "Sure, I don't have a problem with that. There could be something to the theory. I'm just not completely convinced, but I'd like to see this through. I'll write the prescription and we'll see what happens."

"Thank you!" I felt tears prick at the corner of my eyes.

"However, before I give you the prescription, I'd like you to bring him into the office for a rapid strep test. I'll give him the antibiotics either way, but we do need to document this."

The earliest I could get him there was noon the next day. I picked him up from his swimming lesson. I needed to focus all my attention on Joshua, so I asked Kim to stay home with Sydney and Noah.

"Why are we going to Dr. Trish again?" Joshua asked.

"Well, I think you might have some bacteria making your golden circles worse. Dr. Trish has a test for you to take. No shots," I reassured him.

We parked and rode the elevator to the third floor. As we walked down the long corridor he stopped several times to twist his leg.

"What's this?" I asked.

"It's a new one," he said.

Great! I thought.

We didn't have to wait long, fortunately. The medical assistant took Joshua's temperature, which was normal. "What brings you here today?" she asked.

"We're here for the rapid strep test," I said.

She looked at Joshua. "Does your throat hurt?"

"No," he answered.

She looked at me with a puzzled expression.

I sighed. "It's a long story. Dr. Trish knows all about it."

She smiled and swabbed his throat. "It won't take long," she said before leaving the room.

I stood up and walked around the room as we waited for the results. Joshua climbed up on the examination table and scooted onto the window ledge. I was leaning against the wall beside the closed door. I closed my eyes and prayed.

"It's positive," I heard someone say. I heard footsteps and paper shuffling.

"What? Did she have titers run?" I recognized Mindy's voice.

Everything stopped for a moment. *Were they talking about Joshua's results? Maybe someone else is running a test. No, it's got to be Joshua's test. She knew I wanted the titers.*

I looked at Joshua from across the room. His figure was blocking the sun. I remember seeing his small frame silhouetted against the window. I heard his voice, but couldn't process the sound. I felt like I was in a movie, where the room was spinning around me.

If this test is positive, that changes everything!

Chapter Fifteen

I t's positive," Mindy said. "His strep test is positive."

"Oh, really?" I didn't know what else to say.

She turned to Joshua. "How are you feeling, Joshua?"

I had to stop myself from answering, *His throat feels fine. He has no fever, just the anxiety, rage, tics, obsessions, sleeplessness and complete lack of ability to sit still that seems to give us some trouble.* I didn't say a word and waited for Joshua to answer.

"I feel fine," he said at the same time an explosion of facial tics hit.

Mindy chucked. "Now that's a weird look."

"That's the tics," I whispered.

"Oh," she replied, a little embarrassed.

I realized that she didn't really know Joshua at all, despite having seen him in the office since birth. *Did anyone really understand what we were going through?*

"Let me see your throat," she said. Joshua opened his mouth and stuck out his tongue. "Hmm, looks good. OK, pull up your shirt so I can see your belly." She looked perplexed to find nothing there. She checked his bottom, finding no rash there as well.

"Well, Omnicef worked last time. Let's go for that again," she said, handing me the prescription.

"Great. I'll call you next week and let you know how it's going."

"Yes, please do that."

I fought back the tears on the way to the car. I carefully typed Manish a text message, "Joshua tested positive for strep. Going to get the antibiotic now!"

"Mom?"

"Yes, Buddy?"

"Am I sick?"

"Yes."

"What's wrong with me?"

"You just need some antibiotics for a throat infection."

"But my throat doesn't hurt."

"I know, Joshua. It's hard to explain, but if I'm right, in a couple of days, you'll be feeling much, much better. I think this infection might be what's causing all those tics and stuff."

I turned on the radio and called Nani. "Mom, it's positive for strep!"

"You're kidding!"

"No, it's true."

"Does his throat hurt?"

"Nope!"

"Wow!"

"Mom, I think this is it. I think this is the problem. We're on our way to get the prescription now. I have to go now, but I'll call you later."

"Call me tonight, OK?"

"Definitely. Bye, Mom!"

As we walked to the pharmacy, Joshua stopped every six or seven steps to twist his leg. I pushed him along, eager to get him started. We waited fifteen minutes for them to fill the antibiotic. *We've been waiting over two years, what's another fifteen minutes*, I thought.

We walked around the store, looking at things while we waited. Joshua did his six steps, leg twist, six steps, leg twist. People were watching, but I didn't care. Not this time. I picked up the package and gave him the first dosage on the spot, along with a prayer and a hug. *This is it!*

Manish called me as I was driving home. "His test was positive?"

"Yes. I just gave him his first dose of antibiotics. We're on our way home now."

"Good! Very good."

"Manish, I think this is it. I really do."

"Don't get your hopes up. Not yet. Let's just wait and see."

I could tell by his tone that he was excited, but trying to remain the cautious voice of reason.

Friday nights were often movie nights. That night I put on "Monster's Inc.", while I made spaghetti with sauce. The kids loved this movie, even though they'd seen it several times.

I called Manish as I was cooking. "Are you driving home yet?"

"Almost," he replied.

"Good," I said. "I miss you." After the cruise we were much closer. I found the long days without my husband harder to deal with.

"Me, too. How's Joshua doing?"

"It's too early to tell, but they're all watching 'Monster's Inc.' right now."

"Good plan. He'll leave Sydney alone if that movie's on."

"I really think this will work."

"Time will tell!"

"I was thinking that we could count the tics. See if there's progress."

"That's a good idea. Let's see, there's the bird call," Manish said. The bird call was a name we had for a vocal tic of his.

"There's the hawk eye," I said. That's the one where he turns his head, rolling his eyes, while grimacing. "And the lip smacking."

"Yeah, and don't forget the clicks."

"And the new leg thing."

"Right. I'll be home before too long." He hung up and I went back to cooking.

He came home just as I was draining the noodles. He gave me a kiss on the cheek and we exchanged smiles. He went in to watch the movie with the kids. I joined him, looking for a good point to pause.

I've learned that if I stop the movie at the wrong time, dinner could be a very unpleasant experience. Looking at the screen, I could see that Sully had just been banished to the Himalayan Mountains with Mike, the oddball monster. Sully was looking for the little human girl, desperate to get her back. Mike, however, had had enough and didn't want to search through the blizzard for her. He gave his friend an ultimatum, if Sully was going after her, he'd have to do it alone. Sully took off.

I thought this was a good point to pause the movie. "OK, kids, we can watch the rest after dinner!"

Sydney and Noah took their places at the table, while Joshua took his regular seat at the counter. He hadn't been able to eat with us in a while, because he always ended up screaming and crawling under the table.

I usually ate after the kids, not wanting to "choose sides." I hoped that one day we could all eat together, a nice family meal.

I was bustling around the kitchen getting the plates ready for the kids when I noticed that Joshua looked upset. He was very quiet, just watching me. Glancing over at him, I realized he was about to cry.

"Are you OK?" I asked.

"Yeah," he said, looking down.

"What's wrong, Buddy?" It was so rare for him to get tearful about anything.

"Would you do that for me?" he asked, glancing over at the frozen picture on the TV screen. I looked over to see Sully traipsing off into the blizzard after the child.

I wasn't following, but knew this was important to him. "Do what, honey?"

"I mean, would you go all that way, in the snow, for me?" he asked, choking up.

My mouth fell open. My hand froze with the

pasta halfway to the plate, noodles hanging mid-air. "Of course I would, Joshua!" I gasped. I couldn't believe that he'd question that. "I'd do anything for you. Anything. You're my son."

"Really?" he asked, sounding both relieved and excited.

"Yes, Joshua. You're my son. I love you more than life itself. I promise you that I will never stop trying to help you. Ever. No matter what!"

He jumped down from his seat and flew into my arms. "Thank you, Mom!" I hugged him fiercely and continued to whisper words of love to him. I couldn't believe that he didn't know how much I loved him, but I guess through all of this his self-confidence had taken a beating.

Later that night, as was our ritual, I woke him up, so that he could take an extra trip to the bathroom. Before that night, I could always track his progress by his tics. I had the routine memorized. A bird call came before he walked into the bathroom, then the lip smacking kicked in. When he was finished, it was back to the bird call on the return trip to bed. I knew exactly where he was, just by the sounds he was making.

This night was different. I was waiting for him to return from his trip to the bathroom, but there was no narration, no sounds.

It was only when he crawled back into bed with me that I caught a very faint bird call, before he drifted back to sleep. I sat straight up and looked over at him lying there. *No way have the antibiotics worked that fast. It's been less than 24 hours!* I held myself back from waking him again.

The next morning he woke up and the house was silent. I followed him around as he got dressed and prepared for the day. Not one tic!

I gave it some time. *Where's my tic tally list?* I thought. I asked Joshua to pick up his clothes and toys. No tics. Nothing! He was completely silent.

I was so excited I ran down the stairs and called my parents. My father picked up. My father was the youngest mission commander in the Vietnam War. Unfortunately, the years of flying aircraft had taken a toll on his hearing.

"Dad, the tics are gone!" I blurted out.

"We're doin' all right. How are you?" he responded. He has a deep Southern accent.

"No, Dad." I tried to enunciate more clearly. "The tics are gone!"

"The kids are gone?" he asked, sounding a little alarmed.

I yelled, "THE TICS ARE GONE!"

There was silence on the other end. I could feel my voice start to shake. "Dad, can you put Mom on?"

"Oh my gosh," he said. "Just a minute." He immediately made his way through the house, hollering for Mom.

Finally I heard her voice. "What? What is it?"

He put her on. "What's going on?"

"Mom, this is it! They're gone. The tics are gone!"

"You have got to be kidding me! I can't believe it!"

"I know! Manish already left and I can't reach him. He's playing racquetball. We'll connect with him at the swimming pool later," I said.

"Does Joshua notice a difference?"

I paused. "I don't know. I didn't ask him. He didn't say anything. I've got to go. I want to watch him some more. This is so exciting!"

I hung up and raced back up the stairs to watch him some more. He was playing with cars. Normally he'd take two cars and crash them into each other, but now he was playing with them on the track, much more calmly.

I watched him for a bit and then asked, "Joshua, have you noticed you haven't had a single tic all morning?"

He stopped playing and stared at me. "Really? I haven't?"

"No," I said.

A big smile crept across his face. "Does that mean that I'm all better?"

I shook my head. "I don't know. But it's a good sign."

"I hope so!"

"It's only the first day. Let's wait and see what happens."

An hour later the tics were back, but my excitement was still there. They had been affected by the antibiotics. There was hope.

We met Manish at a local indoor pool. He took the boys to get changed and I took Sydney. I realized that her swimsuit didn't make it in the bag, so I raced home with her to get it, since our house was only ten minutes away.

We changed at the house and rushed back to the pool. I immediately knew where Joshua was. The tics were like a cowbell, what with the acoustics of an indoor pool.

As Joshua moved around the pool, people turned to watch. I noticed this more than the tics. Children stared openly and adults tried to avert their gaze, as if nothing was odd about the bird-calling little boy.

I often felt like we were something of a freak show, what with all the vocal tics. I had become used to the looks and learned to avoid eye contact. Some days I came close to making an announcement, "Folks, it's just a little noise. Nothing to be alarmed about," but I never did.

After a couple hours, we went home. Sydney and Noah took naps and Manish and Joshua sat down for a game of chess. Manish enjoyed teaching Joshua. It seemed to help Joshua focus.

I thought I'd try counting tics, to see how he was doing. I counted one hundred and thirty-seven in the next eighty minutes. After that I got depressed and stopped.

When Joshua got up to use the restroom, Manish looked over at me. "Give it more time."

Chapter Sixteen

By the following Sunday, Manish really began to believe that we had found the true problem and solution. Our home was much quieter, almost peaceful. Joshua hadn't had a meltdown in three days. He was playing chess with Manish when Sydney came downstairs. Joshua finished his game and asked to go outside. Sydney followed.

I held my breath. *Here we go!* It was the perfect set-up for a fight. I couldn't believe it when I saw them walking around the house looking for bugs together. Joshua was narrating their nature adventure, as Sydney dutifully listened and followed. She turned and flashed me a smile. I smiled back. *She sees that Joshua's different!*

I ran back to get my video camera. "Manish, they're playing together . . . nicely!" I shouted into the living room. I didn't want to miss anything. I filmed from the porch, so as not to disturb the moment.

The entire day was perfect. No behavioral problems at all. I really enjoyed being with my son.

Manish and I did extensive research on antibiotics. We both realized that Augmentin, a powerful penicillin-based antibiotic, would be best for Joshua. The next day I called the pediatrician and requested a change. Dr. Trish approved it immediately.

The day after that, I called Kim from work to check up on Joshua.

"How are things going?" I asked.

"Amazing," she said. "Joshua's so much calmer now."

"How many tics this morning?"

"I counted five."

"Really? That's great!" It had gone from one hundred and thirty-seven tics in eighty minutes to five in three hundred minutes!

"You know it's funny," she said. "I put Noah and Sydney down for a nap and the house was very quiet. I went down to the basement looking for Joshua, because I was a little worried. I stopped at the landing, so he wouldn't see me. Lori, do you know that he was sitting in the middle of the floor building structures with blocks? He had a huge smile on his face and was singing "Kumbaya" to himself. It was beautiful! He's doing great today, Lori."

I thanked her and hung up the phone. I loved the song "Kumbaya." I had sung it frequently in Girl Scouts, but it wasn't until much later that I learned the origin and meaning of the song. "Kumbaya" is a Gullah word. The Gullah are an African American people who live off the coast of South Carolina. I've had many Gullah patients over the years. "Kumbaya" means "come by here."

Joshua was singing, "Lord, come by here", and I do believe He had come by our home. Later that night I talked to Joshua about the song and its special meaning for me.

"How did you know to read that book?" Joshua asked me, as we cuddled.

I squeezed him on the shoulders and said, "I think it was a God thing."

"Did He talk to you with His voice?" he asked excitedly.

"No, not exactly." I looked for the words to describe how God moves, but the words weren't coming.

"Did He make like a gentle breeze, and did you just follow that breeze?" Joshua floated his fingers in the air to demonstrate his idea.

Tears filled my eyes. "Yes, Joshua!" I said. "I don't think there's any better way to say it."

On Thursday Manish forwarded me two text messages. He had been contacting people in the field. One lady from California, who had written a research article on PANDAS, advised us not to take Joshua off antibiotics for at least six weeks.

The other was from a renowned PANDAS specialist in Chicago. He agreed that since Joshua had responded so well, so quickly, that it was probably PANDAS. He also said that since Joshua had been living with this for so long that we probably needed something stronger. He suggested IVIG. I remembered that from my conversation with Dr. Trish.

The next day Joshua was off again . . . badly. He was irritable, and the tics were back. I checked to make sure he hadn't missed a dose of antibiotics.

No, that wasn't it.

By the next evening, Sydney came down with a sore throat and fever of 102°. Manish looked down her throat to confirm what he suspected. "She's got white patches back there. It's strep!" He announced that we should all go on antibiotics. He called it in and picked it up at the pharmacy.

"What's going on?" I asked when he came home.

"Lori, this won't go away with a round of antibiotics. I've been doing some research on this and any exposure to strep will make Joshua worse. In fact, any exposure to any bacteria or virus will create problems for him. He needs IVIG."

I was shocked. Manish was the last person I would have expected to agree that Joshua needed a medical procedure involving a blood product. He believes that the body can heal itself if given the right circumstances.

"I didn't realize the magnitude of the problem. I thought antibiotics would handle things," I said.

"They'll help, but long term he needs something stronger."

"What exactly is IVIG?" I asked.

Manish took a deep breath. "It's the pooled antibodies of about 10,000 people. They spin the blood down, take the antibodies out and freeze-dry them. Then, when it's time to use it, they add fluid and give it intravenously."

"But what exactly does it do then?" I asked.

"Well, it's a bit like what you do when your computer crashes, and you don't know why. What would you do then?"

"I'd restart it."

"That's basically what IVIG does. It kind of 'reboots' the immune system and wipes out 'previously set' antibodies. In the end the body begins producing new antibodies that give the old ones a new, healthy memory," he said.

Since Manish was set on this, I felt more comfortable with it. I spent a few hours that evening researching on the net.

The next day I made the decision to call Dr. B from work and let him know what we'd discovered. I was nervous about the call, not knowing what he'd say. He'd probably disagree with the course of treatment we'd decided upon. But maybe he knew something that could help. I dialed the number, expecting to get the answering machine. Instead, the nurse answered the phone.

"Hello, this is Lori, Joshua's mother."

"Hi! How are you?"

"Good. Listen, I wanted to let Dr. B know that we've discovered that Joshua has something called PANDAS. I wondered if Dr. B might have any experience with that?"

"Oh yes!" she said confidently. "He actually did a 'grand rounds' on that in medical school."

I was stunned into silence. A grand rounds is a talk that medical professionals give one another on various subjects. Should I just hang up the phone now? I couldn't believe that he'd missed this with Joshua. I mean, he had so many of the symptoms.

"Um, great," I finally said. "So, we'd been giving Joshua Zoloft and then he got a strep infection.

We gave him antibiotics, and when he got better we thought it was the psych meds." I was trying to explain what happened as best I could.

"Oh, that happens sometimes," she casually replied.

What? I thought. *That should never happen!* "So, do you know any other tests I can run to confirm it? We've had two documented strep infections, each with exacerbation of symptoms."

"Hang on, he's right here," she said. I could hear him talking in the background. He was apparently standing right there. *Why don't you just pick up the phone and talk to me?*

"Dr. B says you'll need to run two tests."

"Thanks. I'll need a requisition for them."

"He'll fax it all over for you."

I hung up and went over to my director's office. I plopped down in the chair next to her desk.

"What's wrong?" she asked.

"My psychiatrist wrote a grand rounds paper on PANDAS, but completely missed it with Joshua who'd had nineteen out of twenty of the symptoms," I said in complete disbelief.

"I'd fire him," Laura shot back.

I couldn't believe it. All I could do was sit there. I thought about something my mother had said to me. "Never burn bridges. You might need them."

I heard the fax machine ring. I picked up the form, looking it over. Under the diagnosis area there was nothing but numbers. I knew from my office experience that these were ICD-9 codes, numbers the insurance companies used to determine which procedures receive reimbursement.

Fortunately, we had a book of ICD-9 codes and I could look up the recommendation. The first was strep. That works. Next was Tourette's and the third was OCD. From my research I knew that if Joshua was diagnosed with Tourette's, the insurance company would never pay for IVIG.

I had an appointment with Dr. B in two weeks. I almost cancelled it, but decided against it. I had the feeling I might need something from him.

I had a follow-up appointment with Dr. Trish scheduled. I realized that her foresight of ordering the rapid strep test was brilliant, because now we had another documented case of strep in Joshua's records.

They tested again for rapid strep and it came back negative.

I looked sullenly at her. "I don't want to take him off the antibiotics."

"Augmentin isn't a good long-term one, though," she said. "Azithromycin would be safer. How's he doing?"

"Well, in a word, incredible. Everyone that is with him notices the changes. He is no longer violent. We don't have rages. He doesn't attack his sister. Not to mention the tics are gone."

"That's great."

"Yeah, it was the strep."

"I don't know," she said. "You had him on a lot of Zoloft, too."

"We're weaning him off that now. I read that children with PANDAS can have some really scary reactions with psychiatric medications, especially Zoloft and Haldol."

"I didn't know that," she said.

"What about IVIG?" I asked. "Manish and I would like to give that a try."

"It's actually very safe and I do feel comfortable recommending it, but you'll need to get someone to order it. If you can, I'll help you out. I have a connection that can provide IVIG. I'll write on Joshua's chart that we *discussed* PANDAS," she said. She gave me the number of her contact and she left the room quickly.

As I was driving off I thought about her position. She has to be cautious, and follow the FDA guidelines carefully or her practice could blow up. I realized that I never did get the prescription for the new antibiotic.

I called the office and spoke to Mindy. She gave me the needed dose to prevent reinfection, but said they couldn't call it in. Fortunately, Manish could, so he wrote the prescription. We were set for the next six weeks. Now we had to get the IVIG underway before the antibiotics were up.

Overall, many things had improved with Joshua, but there were still hints of anger. The journey wasn't over. His academic skills had slowly returned, which thrilled him. He was back to improving in math on a daily basis now.

One day I was working with him on a set of math problems.

"I hated it when I couldn't do these," he confided to me.

"I know, Buddy."

"I mean, I was on long division and then I couldn't add two numbers together."

"I just wish that PANDAS would go to some other family and leave us alone," I burst out.

Joshua immediately grabbed my hand and said, "Mom, no! Don't ever say that." He looked into my eyes intently. "I don't want any other little kid to ever have this. Ever! I wish it would just go away from everyone."

I nodded. "You're right."

"Do you remember when Dr. B said that I was waking up because of anxiety?"

"Yes," I said, reorganizing books on the table.

"It wasn't that," he said, as he continued his math.

I realized that Joshua had been aware of all our conversations, during all those appointments. "What was it then?" I leaned on my elbows on the table.

"It was the snakes."

"The WHAT?" I asked, staring at him. "What snakes?"

"When I was four I was really scared of them. They'd be all over the room. But when I was five I learned to jump over them."

"Oh, Joshua!" I said, horrified. "But you know there weren't really snakes in your room, right?"

He looked at me with a shocked expression. "Of course they were real. They were all black and slithery. Rattlesnakes make noise before they bite. These snakes didn't look like rattlesnakes, but they made the noise. That's why I was afraid they were going to bite me."

"Why didn't you tell me?"

"I don't know. I just couldn't. They were mostly in my room, but they also came to your room if I spent the night there. Not as many though. That's why I liked to sleep there better."

Suddenly, I began to understand some of his nightly rituals a little better. "They weren't in the basement, were they?"

"Right, no snakes in the basement. That's why I liked to sleep down there. It was one of the few places where I was safe."

I pulled him into my arms. "I'm so sorry, Joshua. I had no idea." On top of everything, he'd been hallucinating and I didn't even know it. "Do you still see the snakes?"

"No," he said. "They went away when you gave me the medicine from Dr. Trish."

"I'm so glad," I said, hugging him tightly. I rocked him back and forth. *I'll get you the treatment you need, Joshua. I promise you that you'll never have to go back to that reality again.*

Chapter Seventeen

There are moments in life that you never forget. You remember exactly where you were, what the air smelled like, what was around you. In this journey there have been a few such moments for me. Moments where the world just stopped, where I knew something big had just happened.

One of these times was when I had just left a patient's house in rural Missouri. My cell phone rang. I saw it was Manish, so I pulled over on a gravel road next to a big round silo.

"Did you talk to Dr. Trish's contact?" I asked without preamble.

"Yes. He agreed to order the IVIG for Joshua."

I released the breath I had been holding. "That's great news!"

"Only catch is, they need a letter saying that Joshua has PANDAS and that IVIG is an acceptable treatment," he said. There was worry in his voice.

Oh, come on, we've come so close! "Can't you just write it?" I asked.

"No," he answered flatly. "It has to come from a pediatric specialist."

"Why won't anyone help us?" I cried. "This is crazy!"

"Calm down," he said. His strong voice was reassuring. "He needs this. We'll do what we have to, to get it done."

"But what if we can't find someone?"

"Then we'll drive to Chicago and see the specialist there. It will cost $20,000, and the insurance won't cover it, but it's just money. Joshua's health is more important. We'll find a way."

"We shouldn't have to do that, though," I said. "This is ridiculous."

"I agree. Why won't Dr. Trish write it again?"

"She's not willing to actually give him the diagnosis of PANDAS," I reminded him.

"Right," he said. "OK, so who else is there? Who else do we know that could write the letter?"

"Dr. B."

"Oh, and he's been a *great* help!"

"I know, but he's really our only chance." I gave a silent prayer of thanks that I had followed my mother's advice and not burned that bridge. There was hope.

"Do you think he'll do it?" Manish asked.

"Yes, he will. I'll call him right away and start bugging him."

"Do you want me to call?"

I laughed. "No, I don't think that's a good idea. You're bound to lose your temper. Then where will we be? Let me deal with him, OK?"

I hung up with Manish and called the office. I got the machine and asked Dr. B to call me back about Joshua's treatment.

It was 6:00 p.m. when the nurse called me back.

The kids were all screaming in the background, so I spoke quickly. I explained how badly we needed it, going over the difficulties we were having. She seemed surprised that we were having so much trouble and assured me that they could certainly write it. She asked me to type up an e-mail with all the pertinent information, so that she could make sure the letter was written.

I got off the phone, put the kids to bed and started working on the letter. When I finished, I crawled into bed. "I think we have our letter!"

"I'll believe it when we have it in hand," Manish mumbled.

"Don't worry. We'll get it."

The next day, no letter. Next day, no letter. Finally, on Friday morning I called the office and left a message. Friday afternoon the secretary called to let me know that they didn't get the e-mail.

I should have called earlier, I thought, mentally kicking myself. I just didn't want to bug them too much. I still had an appointment with Dr. B set for Monday, so I realized my best shot was to see him in person and get the letter then. Maybe Dr. B wanted to see him one more time before ordering IVIG, hence the delay.

Joshua was having difficulty again. We had switched the antibiotic to Amoxicillin, deciding that the Azithromycin wasn't working. I prayed that Dr. B didn't take one look at him and decide it wasn't PANDAS.

I realized that it wouldn't hurt if I wrote a letter for Dr. B to sign. It would be easier for him. He could just sign it on Monday and be done with it. I researched what the letter should state and how it should be worded. I showed it to Manish, who agreed it was perfect.

On Sunday night I thought to call a close family friend, an experienced pharmacist. She explained that Azithromycin was way overused, so it wasn't nearly as effective as it once was. She also felt that Amoxicillin was too weak. We revisited the dosage and talked to Manish about going back on Augmentin. He agreed, and called the prescription in to the local drugstore.

It was too late to pick it up that night, so I had to wait until the next morning. I hoped that giving Joshua a dose before the appointment with Dr. B would work out. Given the right antibiotic, the reaction was fast.

I didn't sleep well that night, worrying about the next day. Bleary-eyed, I stumbled into the store at 8:00 a.m. with Joshua in tow.

"I'm here to pick up a prescription for Joshua Suthar," I told the young college guy behind the counter.

He typed in his name and shook his head. "Nothing here for anyone by that name."

I'd had it. I was exhausted and tired of no one helping us, fighting against the world to save my son. Unfortunately for this young man, he seemed to be standing in the way of my son's treatment, so he received the brunt of my anger.

"Check the computer again!" I barked at him, strongly considering jumping over the counter and finding the Augmentin myself.

He typed it in again and shook his head. "No, nothing here." This time he looked a little apologetic and somewhat afraid.

"Did you bother to check the messages this morning?" I asked, realizing that my voice sounded snide. I could see the pharmacist in the background picking up the phone to check. I knew the message was there, because I'd been standing by Manish's side when he phoned it in.

While I waited, Joshua had escaped and returned with a bag of crackers. "Could I have this Mom?"

"Sure," I said, not taking my eye off the pharmacist on the phone.

Normally, I would never allow my children to open a bag in the middle of a store, but I knew he hadn't eaten and would need something in his stomach for the medication. I acted as if it were completely normal.

"Can I get something to drink?"

"Sure," I said flatly. I was too exhausted to put up any argument. "Why not?"

I'm sure he thought he'd won the lottery. He swiftly came back with a bottle of grape juice. He handed it to me and I opened it, still staring down the pharmacist.

"There was one message left late last night," the pharmacist said.

"That's it!" I said. "That would be our prescription."

His ears were turning red. The Augmentin was

ready in record time. He took the bag of crackers in order to scan them, but grabbed it too fast, causing crackers to fly in all directions.

We left quickly, much to the relief of the staff. In the parking lot I gave Joshua his dosage. *Please let it absorb into his body quickly*, I prayed.

I got home, picked up the letter for Dr. B and got ready for the appointment.

"What are you going to do if he backs out and doesn't agree to sign?" Manish asked.

I gave him a determined smile. "Bring cash to work in case you have to bail me out of jail for assault, OK?"

Chapter Eighteen

As I drove Joshua to Dr. B's office I ran through all the scenarios in my mind. I tried to anticipate all of his possible objections, although, to date, he'd given none. I still wanted to be prepared.

I'll give him the letter to sign first, I thought. *I need to get him to fax it over, but I want to keep the original. How am I going to explain that?*

I parked and read over the letter I'd written, as I sat in the car. I'm not sure why, as I couldn't change it if there were an error.

August 23, 2010

Dear Dr. I,

Joshua Suthar has a diagnosis of PANDAS (Pediatric Autoimmune Neuropsychiatric Disorder Associated with Strep). IVIG is an appropriate treatment intervention. The following is from the NIMH website regarding IVIG:

Q: What about treating PANDAS with plasma exchange or immunoglobulin (IVIG)?

A: The results of a controlled trial of plasma exchange (also known as plasmapheresis) and immunoglobulin (IVIG) for the treatment of children in the PANDAS subgroup was published in "The Lancet", Vol. 354, October 2, 1999. All of the children participating in the study had clear evidence of a strep infection as the trigger of their OCD and tics, and all were severely ill at the time of treatment. The study showed that plasma exchange and IVIG were both effective for the treatment of severe, strep triggered OCD and tics, and that there were persistent benefits of the interventions.

Current dosage for PANDAS is 1.5g/kg over a period of 2 days.

I had typed Dr. B's name and left room for him to sign. It looked good.

"Mom?" Joshua asked.

"Yeah?"

"Are we going in?"

"Yeah, Buddy. I'm ready," I said.

I walked into Dr. B's office with my plan, but we ended up talking first for a while. I didn't want to press my luck. I told him how bad the symptoms had gotten.

Dr. B glanced over at Joshua, looking shocked. I grinned, realizing that the last time he'd seen my son, Joshua had been upside down on the couch and digging bugs out of the windowsill. Today he was sitting cross legged, putting together a puzzle on the floor.

I went over the research I'd done, pretending that I didn't know about the grand rounds paper. I went over how Joshua tested positive to strep and how well he'd done on the antibiotics.

Then I finally handed him the letter. *Please sign it*, I silently pleaded.

He read it over and nodded. "Looks fine. I'll

have the secretary type it up and send it over."

NO, I screamed in my head. *That won't work. I'm not leaving until it's faxed and I have a copy.*

As if he'd read my mind, he glanced at the letter again and said, "Actually, it looks fine how it is. You did a good job." He slid it into Joshua's folder. It was then that I noticed that he had doodled "PANDAS" on the outer cover.

He escorted Joshua and me out to the receptionist where I'd pay for the visit. I never took my eyes off Joshua's file.

"Actually," I said bravely, "would you mind faxing it now? See, I'd like to keep the original." I laughed, madly thinking of a reason that might make sense. Finally I blurted out, "Some parents keep their children's artwork for their scrapbooks. Joshua's scrapbook is filled with doctor's letters and evaluations." I held my breath. Would it work?

He shrugged his shoulders. "Sure," he said. He quickly signed the letter, before sliding it into the fax machine.

I waited the agonizing minute it took to fax the document to the doctor's office and then put out my hand to receive the letter back. He complied, and I raced out of the office as fast as I could, just in case he changed his mind.

I called Manish. "It's done. The letter's faxed and I have a copy!"

"Wow, you're incredible! Well done!"

"Thanks! Can you call to set up the appointment?"

"Sure, I'll do it this afternoon," he promised.

I couldn't wait that long. "Don't worry, I'll do

it."

He chuckled. "Good idea."

I looked up the number on my cell phone and called from the parking lot.

"What does tomorrow look like, Mrs. Suthar?" the girl on the other end asked.

"Wow, that's fast!" I said. "Tomorrow's great!" I had no idea what we had scheduled for tomorrow, but it didn't matter. This took priority over everything.

"Morning or afternoon?" she asked casually.

"Morning." *The sooner the better.*

I hung up and sat down. His first IVIG appointment was scheduled for August 24, 2010, one month and one day after he tested positive for strep.

Chapter Nineteen

After the kids had gone to bed, I walked into Manish's office and sat on the edge of his desk. "We're set for tomorrow," I said.

He looked up at me in surprise. "That fast?"

"Yeah," I said with a smile.

"I wonder what it's going to cost."

"Probably less than Chicago."

"I hope so, that's $20,000," Manish said.

"Too bad we can't find a way to get my insurance to cover it."

Since Manish was in private practice, health insurance was ridiculously expensive. When I started working part time, I was offered a limited benefit plan. It was pretty good and a strong incentive to keep that job.

"They don't cover PANDAS," Manish said, dismissing the idea.

"I know. But I can always hope!"

The next morning I woke up nauseous. *Would this be it?*

We ate breakfast. It was important that Joshua eat something, because of all the medication he was on. It didn't do well on an empty stomach.

I had explained everything to Joshua at home. Manish and I make a point of never sugar-coating the truth. As a result, Joshua always knows that we'll be straight with him.

As we walked into the cancer center Joshua asked, "When do I get my needle?"

"Soon, Buddy," I said. "First I have to do some paperwork."

We walked down the hallway and entered the children's suite. I was amazed. It was covered with baseball decorations. There was an arcade, a Wii, toys, games and a slurpee machine. It was a dream for any child. Joshua wanted to run into the room and start playing, but I asked him to stay with me, while I took care of the forms.

The young receptionist handed me a clipboard with all the basic paperwork. "I called the insurance company and you don't need a precertification. You should be fine."

"What do you mean?" I asked.

"They should pay," she said.

I stood motionless, with the clipboard frozen midair. *Close your mouth, Lori*, I thought, as I realized my jaw was hanging down to the ground. *Say something!*

Finally I said, "I thought there wasn't an ICD-9 code for PANDAS. How can they pay?"

"Oh," she said with a smile. "PANDAS causes encephalitis, so that's how we code it."

She was right. Encephalitis is an inflammation in the brain, which causes these symptoms. I couldn't believe it. Was it possible that we wouldn't have to pay anything for these visits?

"I'll stay on it and let you know," she said.

I took the clipboard and sat down next to Joshua. He was being very cooperative, knowing that the second I finished the forms he could go and play. I gave him permission to look through the cabinets, just as long as he stayed within my field of vision.

A young nurse, Jamie, came over to me. "I have some cream to numb his arm. Is that OK?"

"Sure," I answered. I became excited. *It's really going to happen. We did it!*

She called Joshua over and began applying the cream. "It has to sit for a while before it's numb," she explained, as she put gauze over it. "I'll come back when it's time."

"How many children have you treated for PANDAS?" I asked.

"Joshua will be our third," she answered with a smile.

"How did the other kids do?"

"Well, one was fourteen years old. I think he needed two treatments, but he's doing well now."

"That's great," I said. "I've read that after puberty, the chances of success are reduced."

"Yes, it's good that your son is young. You caught it early."

"I can't tell you how grateful we are for this solution," I said.

Jamie smiled at me. "The dosage your doctor ordered is high. I'm a little puzzled that there haven't been any other blood tests ordered."

"What other tests?" I asked nonchalantly. I didn't tell her that I knew the dosage because my husband and I had consulted with the world specialist for PANDAS and that this was his protocol. I also didn't mention that I had written the needed letter.

"ASO titers or immune function tests."

"He's here because of his strep history."

"Makes sense," she said.

She left the room and ten minutes later the IVIG specialist came in, introducing himself. He sat down and addressed Joshua directly. "How are you feeling?"

At that moment Joshua had a burst of facial tics.

"How long has that been going on?" he asked.

"About a year," Joshua answered casually.

"Well, let's see if we can't help you with that."

Twenty minutes later Jamie came in. "OK, Joshua, we're ready for you!"

We went into a small room, with a TV, a few toys and an examining table. She asked for the list of medications that Joshua was taking, with the doses.

I could feel Joshua's anxiety rising, as he anticipated the needle stick. Jamie sensed it too and called in another nurse to help her. They slid the needle in quickly.

"Wow, that didn't even hurt!" Joshua said, exhaling loudly.

"That's good, Buddy," I said, stroking his hair.

I figured out the TV system while Jamey started the IV. I found a cartoon that Joshua liked and he settled in on the table.

"How long will this last?" I asked.

"About 4-5 hours."

I hadn't anticipated it going that long. I called my father-in-law, asking if he could bring lunch. At noon he walked in with Joshua's favorite fast food meal, chicken nuggets and apple juice. Manish came in shortly after, eager to see how Joshua was progressing.

The next morning I woke Joshua a bit earlier, in order to feed him a good breakfast. He wasn't hungry.

I groaned. "Come on, Buddy. You've got to eat!"

"I don't feel well."

"I know, Honey. It's just important to eat something when you take these medicines."

"OK, Mom," he said. "How about a yogurt tube?"

"That'll work." In the end I got him to eat a few walnuts, too.

They had given me the numbing cream, so that he could be ready upon arrival. I quickly applied it.

Joshua was quiet on the twenty minute ride to the hospital. I glanced back at him in the rearview mirror. He looked pale. "Buddy, are you all right back there?"

"I think I'm going to throw up," he said just as we were pulling into the hospital parking lot.

He didn't eat enough before he took the Augmentin, I thought. I grabbed an empty bag sitting on the front seat and handed it back to him. "Here, use this if you need it."

He got out of the van, clutching the bag, looking at the ground. He just stood outside for a moment. After taking a few deep breaths he said, "I can make it. Let's go."

I smiled as I ushered him through the doors. He was becoming such a mature guy, willing to face anything. I couldn't imagine going through this with any other child.

As soon as we entered the cancer center, I grabbed a trash bin and sat him down. "Just in case," I said. "I'll be right back." I checked us in and went back to the kitchen area. Inside the refrigerator were juice boxes for the patients. I took two.

Joshua downed the first one quickly, much to my relief. I had read that hydration goes a long way toward helping the side effects.

They stuck his arm again. This time the needle didn't want to go in. It took four nurses, but finally it went in and we settled down for another four hours.

They had marvelously heated blankets that Joshua loved. They brought new ones every thirty minutes or so.

"I don't want to watch TV anymore," he said after a few hours.

"OK, Buddy. No problem." I turned the television off.

The room was silent.

"Is the PANDAS gone?" he asked.

"I sure hope so!" I replied.

"Me too."

"The medicine will get rid of it."

He closed his eyes and was quiet for a while. I pulled out my electronic reader and selected a novel to read. Nothing medical, just pure pleasure. Joshua's soft voice startled me. "Mom?"

"Yeah, Buddy?"

"My sixth year was horrible."

"I know. I know."

"I can't ever be six again." Tears were welling up in his eyes. "I can't ever get that year back".

I choked back my tears. It was important that I stay strong. "We did have some good times, too, you know."

He opened his eyes and stared at the ceiling. "Yeah, but I was sad and you were even more sad." He had a way of cutting straight to the point.

"You're right. It has been a hard year for us all. Especially you." I stood up and stroked his arm. "You know what?"

He looked at me. "What?"

"Seven is going to be awesome!"

"Yeah!"

"You know we're pretty blessed to have this treatment," I said. "Jamey was telling me about a boy who didn't find out he had PANDAS until he was fourteen years old!"

"That's horrible," he cried.

"I know."

This was the Joshua I knew years ago, my deep thinker. We sat in silence and I began thinking of how my own faith had grown. I had learned how to pray when I had no words. I had finally learned that "peace that passes all understanding," something people had so flippantly said since I was a little girl.

I no longer had a shred of belief in coincidence or fate. I knew something amazing would come from this. This experience had changed me and Joshua as well. People always say that circumstances make you who you are. I don't believe that anymore either. I believe that circumstances "reveal" who we are.

If someone had told me that our family would go through this, I would have been petrified. Faith had brought us through and now I know how to depend on it.

Joshua has the blessing of learning this at such a young age. He often asks, "How did you know to keep me at home even before the PANDAS got so bad?" Sometimes he asks, "Isn't it amazing that Dr. Trish knew someone at the cancer center that could help us when no one else could?" or "How did you find that book, Saving Sammy, again?"

He knows now that things don't happen by chance or luck, they are orchestrated, and we may never really know the impact of our experiences.

He thought for a moment. "Do you think there are more kids out there that have this and don't know it? Why don't their doctors help them?"

Good question, I thought. "Well, a lot of doctors don't know about PANDAS. And the ones that have heard about it don't always believe it."

"What? Why?"

"I don't have a good answer to that, Buddy."

"Well, we should tell them," he said matter-of-factly.

It was then that I thought about writing a book about this experience. "Maybe we should," I said. "It would be worth it if we could help just one child."

Chapter Twenty

L unch time rolled around and I talked Joshua into going down to the cafeteria. They didn't have a lot to offer, but I did manage to interest Joshua in a few pieces of chicken and a soda.

During lunch the IV pole started beeping. Joshua and I looked at each other and said, "That's it!"

It was over. Our two day miracle was over.

We got home and went to bed early. Joshua and I were beyond exhausted.

The next day we had a picnic with his new school, which would start in a little less than two weeks. Manish and I decided it was worth going, as he'd most likely meet some of his new classmates. Plus, a little sun and fresh air sounded good.

Joshua immediately took off with the kids his age, befriending a boy that would be in his class. I watched him – no tics! And Sydney ran off to join in a game of hide-and-seek. *So this is what it's like to be a normal family*, I thought.

About thirty minutes after dinner Joshua's eyes started to droop. We packed everyone up and headed home.

I walked in the door and began preparing his

medicine.

"Mom?" he cried.

I turned to look at him. "What is it, Buddy?"

"My head hurts!" he was crying. "It's beating, Mom. It hurts!"

I got him to swallow the medicine and added in a pain reliever. He was unable to stand, so I carried him into our bedroom.

As horrible as that sounds, it was a great sign. I had read that massive headaches are a very positive sign that the IVIG is working. It was rough to see him in so much pain, but I knew it was short-term. He was on the mend.

Joshua buried himself under the covers and I climbed in next to him. I'd never seen him in so much pain.

"Honey, this is the medicine working. The PANDAS is going away."

"Mom, get closer to me," he said.

I held him and whispered, "I love you, Joshua."

We stayed that way for a little while. He moaned quietly, but didn't move a muscle.

"Stay with me," he pleaded.

"I'm not going anywhere, sweetheart. I'll be here as long as you need me."

"All night?"

"All night."

I fell asleep quickly. Manish looked in on us throughout the night. The next morning he told me that Joshua hadn't fallen asleep until 5:00 a.m.

I had a patient in the morning, so I called one of my babysitters. I promised Joshua that I would return with food from his favorite restaurant, and lemonade. I saw a few patients that day, coming back to see Joshua in-between visits. By the afternoon he was feeling better and moved to the couch.

Over the next few days I spent countless hours on the internet looking for what to expect, what other parents had observed in their PANDAS children.

Some had miracles right in the IVIG room, but the majority reported significant changes within three or four months. Some needed a second treatment.

I started ticking off the days on the calendar. The first two weeks didn't go well. In fact, they were the worst in two years. Joshua's voice took on a weird tone when he got angry, which was often. He'd also reverted to baby talk, something I hadn't seen before.

One evening he was trying to do a puzzle. He was becoming increasingly frustrated as he had more and more trouble putting the pieces together. I tried to help, but he just became more agitated. When I reached to put the puzzle away, I felt a sharp pain on my knuckles. Joshua had thrown a remote across the room.

I asked Sydney to take Noah downstairs. We both knew what was going to happen. As soon as they left Joshua launched his body against me and began attacking. I was prepared and subdued him quickly.

"This is not you," I reminded him quietly.

"Get off me!" he screamed. He was straining with all his might, sweating against me.

This time was different. I knew there was a light at the end of the tunnel, which helped me remain calm. Soon he calmed down, so I set him up to watch television in my room. He laid his head on the pillow and allowed the cartoon to lull him to sleep. *We have a little over a week to get you ready for school*, I thought as I watched his quiet breathing.

A few nights later he came running out of his room a couple hours after he went to bed. "I'm scared," he cried out.

"I'm coming," I called as I raced up the stairs. *At least I know what's going on now*. When I reached his room I pushed open the door. "Is it the snakes?" I asked, a little out of breath.

"No," he said quietly. He slowly turned around with a scared look on his face. "I just keep feeling like there are people walking behind me." His eyes seemed to follow invisible targets around the room.

"How about if I leave the door open and then –"

"No!" he shouted. He ran and closed the door behind me. "More will just come in if you do that."

"OK," I said casually. "How about if we figure out what you'll wear tomorrow?" Maybe that would be a simple distraction.

"Leave the closet door closed," he said firmly.

I stopped and turned to him. "Would you like to sleep with me in the basement?" By this time I was completely freaked out and didn't want to spend another minute in this room. It seemed haunted.

"Yes," he said relieved. "That would be great."

The next day I showed Joshua a catalogue with new sheets, comforter, curtains and decorations. We went together to the paint store and picked out the colors for his room.

I couldn't erase the memories of the last year, but I could certainly make his room a safe haven for him. The old one had too many bad memories, filled with slithery snakes and invisible people. I wanted to get rid of it all.

Chapter Twenty-One

Day by day the tics lessened. I wasted an enormous amount of time just watching him do everyday things, things he couldn't do a few months ago. We continued to wean him off the Zoloft and Strattera. It was a slow process.

Our school started a little later than the other local schools. I chose to take advantage of the extra time and take the three kids to the Science Center, something I would have never attempted by myself previously.

When we entered the children's area, I held my breath. Six months ago Joshua had almost completely demolished a teepee display. He now chose to color a picture at a work station, along with a few other children. The picture was beautiful.

He then politely asked one of the employees for assistance with a musical instrument. I reminded myself that I needed to keep an eye on the two younger children as well. Sydney was playing with a Madagascar hissing cockroach, while Noah was happily pressing buttons on a computer.

I sat down in complete disbelief, allowing myself to breathe normally for the first time in a long while. We were going to make it. School started in less than a week and we were going to be OK!

When I got home later that day, I looked at the calendar and sighed. I'd completely forgotten we'd signed Joshua up for tryouts for the swim team at the local gym a few months ago. I learned about the swim team through a friend whose child has autism. Her son never really competed, but he enjoyed practicing a lot. We had thought Joshua would like it, too.

When I'd signed him up I hadn't known about IVIG. Joshua was improving rapidly, but I thought this might be a bit much. He still was regaining his energy.

At the dinner table I brought the subject up. "Tryouts for the swim team are tomorrow. I'm thinking we should wait until next time."

"No, Mom. Please?" he begged. "I really want to try."

I looked to Manish. I didn't want him to miss out on this, but I didn't want to push him.

"I think it's fine," Manish said, shrugging his shoulders.

I smiled. "OK, Joshua, we'll go as planned."

"Yay! Thanks, Mom!"

Manish agreed to stay home with the other kids, so that I could devote my energy to watching Joshua in the pool. When we arrived there were about fifty children of all ages ready to try out.

I registered him, helped him change and headed over to the waiting room. It had a large glass window, so I could watch him.

The kids were all lined up on the far wall.

Joshua, being extremely excited, sat down at the edge of the pool and dangled his feet in the shallow end. He hadn't noticed the other children, so he did what he did every other time he'd come to the pool for swim lessons.

I groaned. He was the only one not sitting on the wall. I couldn't call to him from the glassed-in room, but I tried to motion to him to go to the wall. Something then caught my eye.

A man was motioning wildly from his seat, near me. He was clearly agitated. At first I assumed he was gesturing to his own child, but then I realized he was focused on my son. I heard him say, "The wall! The wall! Sit down at the wall!"

I was infuriated. *Who the hell do you think you are talking to my child that way,* I thought. *This isn't the freaking Olympics, you know. It's the neighborhood gym!*

I looked over at Joshua, who was deep in conversation with the lifeguard, oblivious to this man's comments. The lifeguard knew Joshua and motioned for him to get in the water. When Joshua slid into the shallow end the parent came undone. "Against the wall!" he yelled.

The people in the room began to look around. The kids couldn't hear him, so I'm not sure what this man thought he was going to accomplish.

There have been a very few times in my life when I felt the urge for violence. This was one of them. After all we'd been through this year, here my son was finding joy, and this man wanted to ruin it. I kept myself in check and simply glared hateful beams at the back of his bald, fat head.

Joshua glanced over at the glass room, looking for my face. When he caught my eye he gave me a huge smile, waving excitedly.

I stood up and waved back, giving him the thumbs up sign. I shouted, "Good job!" so that the big ox in front of me could hear. I silently dared him to say anything to me. He didn't even turn around.

One of the teachers took five kids into the water to join Joshua. He had them all bob in the water for a bit and then they started for the other side of the pool. One of the requirements for the swim team was that the child must be able to swim the entire length of the pool.

Joshua had made it about halfway once, but I thought the challenge would be good for him. I didn't expect him to make it all the way, but he knew to swim for the side if he got tired.

Joshua swam and swam, passing the halfway mark. I stood up and watched as he dog paddled his way to the other side. He made it!

I thought he'd get out of the water then, but instead he headed back. I was so proud of him. I never expected him to make it all the way back. I found myself cheering for him, moving closer to the front of the room. When he made it all the way to the other side he turned around, grinning. I waved at him, wildly, nearly jumping up and down.

I ran through the dressing rooms and found him.

"Did you see me?" he cried.

"Of course! I was watching the whole time."

"Did you see that I made it all the way across

the pool and back?"

"You were amazing!" I cried, hugging his wet body.

I helped him to get dressed and then we headed back the way we came. As I was turning in the last of the paperwork, a young man handed me a yellow slip with Joshua's name, age and team name on it.

"You made it, Joshua!" I cried.

"I did?"

"Yeah, it says so right here." I showed him the slip.

"Wow! Let's go home and tell Dad. He won't believe it!"

When we got into the car he asked me if we could call his grandparents. They shouted praises over the phone, causing Joshua to grin from ear to ear.

When we pulled into the garage, Joshua ran out of the car to tell Manish. When I walked in the door, Manish looked at me for confirmation.

"He did it!" I exclaimed proudly. "He swam the entire length of the pool and back. Joshua was extraordinary!"

Manish beamed at him.

Chapter Twenty-Two

A few days before school started I spoke to the office staff. I told the nurse about Joshua's condition, asking her to please notify me the second anyone in Joshua's class had strep. An exposure to strep probably meant another IVIG treatment.

His teacher was very understanding, which put me at ease. She immediately understood the importance of the condition.

The first day of school was very exciting. Joshua put on his uniform shirt and raced down the stairs to join Sydney for breakfast. They both grabbed their backpacks and piled into the car. Noah would be going to the preschool at their school twice a week.

We got there ten minutes early. I gave them both a little pep talk before dropping them off. As I drove off I tried not to worry.

Manish called me throughout the day to check in and see how Joshua was doing. The school hadn't called, so I had nothing to report. I didn't want to be overbearing, so I didn't call them.

I was first in line to pick him up at the end of the day. I saw him and started waving frantically.

His teacher stopped by the car to let me know

that Joshua had done well. She was calm and sounded sincere. I thanked her and ushered the kids into the van. As we pulled away, I bombarded Joshua with questions.

"How did it go? Did you meet any new friends? Did you have any trouble with tics?"

He glared at me. "Don't talk to me!" he screamed.

Uh oh, I thought. *I hope that didn't happen at school.*

I turned back around to Sydney and asked about her day. She smiled and said she had a good time. I glanced back over at Joshua, who had fallen asleep. He was obviously exhausted.

The first two weeks of school were like this. I learned not to talk to him when he got into the car. Within five minutes he was always asleep. I often drove around, allowing him a little extra sleep.

We were careful to put him to bed early, but it still wasn't enough sleep. However, after two weeks things leveled off. His energy level increased.

I signed up to drive his class on their first field trip. I had five second-graders in my van. I watched him interact with the other kids and was pleased to see him smiling and laughing with them, participating in the fun and games. I had never seen that before.

There were a few times when Joshua said something slightly inappropriate. The others were quick to tell him, "If you say something like that again, you'll lose your turn." He caught on quickly. These were his new friends and they were gently giving him an education in being a second grader.

They were the best therapy he'd ever had.

After a few weeks, we were invited to an open house where we could meet all the teachers and see the classrooms. I couldn't wait. I really wanted to talk to Joshua's teacher and find out how he was doing.

I was prepared for the worst, but was thankful that Joshua had at least made it for a few weeks. Manish and I hired a baby sitter, so that we could give our undivided attention to the teachers. We went to Sydney's class first, then Noah's, leaving Joshua's for last.

I took a deep breath before we entered Joshua's classroom. His teacher, Mrs. Feulner, sat down across from us at one of the small desks.

"How's Joshua doing?" I asked, as I sat down. *Might as well get to it.*

"He's doing great!" she replied.

I looked at her, looking for any signs that she was politely holding back anything. Her demeanor indicated that she was sincere.

Manish and I looked at one another. I decided to pry a bit. "How is his behavior?"

"Well, we have a behavior system with cards. Because they are second grade boys, I give them an extra warning before I have them flip cards. Everyone starts with a green, then it flips to blue, then orange. At that point, if it gets to orange, they go to time out," she explained.

"What color's Joshua's card?"

"Oh, I don't think he's flipped a card," she replied.

"Wow, that's great!" I said.

"Yes, he's been really good."

Manish leaned forward. "How about at the beginning of the school year?"

"All children go through something of an adjustment," she said. "But Joshua wasn't out of the ordinary. I'd say he was just about average in that department."

Manish and I looked at each other and smiled.

"Anything we can work on at home?" I asked.

"Handwriting," she said. "We're starting cursive now."

"We can certainly work on that!"

"You know what he loves to do when he has free time?" she asked.

"No, what?" I asked.

"Reading. He really enjoys sitting in the book area and reading."

I felt tears well up in my eyes.

"That's great!" Manish said, standing up. "That's really wonderful to hear."

I followed suit, standing up. We thanked Mrs. Feulner and walked out the door and up the stairs. We were both in a bit of shock, as neither of us had expected a good report.

"I guess he saved the bad behavior during those first two weeks for home," I said.

"Good thing!" Manish replied.

"I'll say."

"He's such a smart boy, even when he's sick."

"I can't believe it, but I think he's actually going to be OK!" I exclaimed as we walked out the door into the fresh air.

Manish put his arm around me, kissing the top of my head. "I think so!"

I looked around at the other parents, walking up and down the front steps of the school, talking about their teacher conferences. I realized that we looked just like them. We did it. Through prayer, persistence and faith, we got our son back.

Epilogue

Last November, some of Joshua's symptoms returned, mainly the clicking. We contacted the specialist in Chicago who reviewed all of Joshua's records, researching his precise situation. In the end, he recommended a second IVIG treatment, which Joshua received a month later.

It was definitely the right call. We saw immediate changes for the better, but the majority of the improvements came about fourteen weeks later. Although it will take a full year for Joshua to heal from the second infusion, he will most likely make a full recovery.

This May, Joshua finished the second grade with A's and B's. He's been wonderfully talkative, making up for lost time. He's an avid swimmer and his math skills are back to Joshua normal. In addition, he participated in a speech contest, something I never thought I'd see a year ago.

Although there is a high incidence of PANDAS affecting siblings, Sydney and Noah have never shown signs. We think that the high dose of penicillin Sydney received in Mexico for strep may have saved her.

We are thankful Joshua was able to get the treatment he so desperately needed, but it haunts me that there are other families dealing with this monstrous illness. It is horrible to see one's child physically before you, yet know that he isn't really there.

The medical professionals who have known Joshua the longest are convinced of the accuracy of his diagnosis. He has PANDAS. Our pediatrician, Dr. Trish, is now extremely supportive and agrees that our son is a completely different child. Since Joshua's successful treatments, Dr. B has directed another parent in testing her child for PANDAS, which turned out to be an accurate diagnosis.

I know of three other families, whose children were diagnosed with OCD, who turned out to have PANDAS. Two of those families have successfully pursued IVIG and had tremendous results. The lives of their children are changed forever. There are likely thousands more children suffering from this disorder at this writing. Unfortunately, the psychiatric community is placing these children on strong medications, which are very dangerous, especially for children with PANDAS.

My hope is that this book may save the lives of other children. When I watch TV and see some child commit a crazy, out of character, violent act or the incidence of autism rise again, I wonder, could there be a connection?

Acknowledgments

I would have never made it through the past few years without the support of my husband and family and the people who help take care of our children.

Manish, I can't believe what we have overcome in our sleepless stupor. You are right, life is so good and only when you have experienced the darker side can you truly appreciate the light.

To my co-writer, Laura Sherman, thank you so much for your patience and for holding my hand through this process. What an amazing author and person you are. I look forward to our next book!

Kim, Shirley, and Marla, your unconditional love and acceptance of Joshua, no matter what, is such a statement of love and faith. I honestly can't imagine going through this without you.

Mom, Dad and Ken, thank you for teaching me how to deal with life and that sometimes it throws you curves. Mom, thanks for reminding me to keep my eyes focused upward and to keep putting my feet on the floor everyday . . . turns out there was a reason I was so stubborn as a child . . . I would need it as a mother.

A sincere thank you to Manish's family for their support, love and acceptance through our ordeal.

Felicia, my sister, when we survive parenthood, we will once again enjoy a nice chai with Belgian chocolate!

Vik, thanks for taking the time to discuss the legal and professional aspects of all of this.

My friends at Community Bible Study, what a support and encouragement you all have been. Special thanks to my Tuesday "prayer warriors" Shelly, Sheryl, Judy, Stephanie, Terri and Annie. Thanks for reminding me to stay on my knees and just being ears and hearts for me and my family.

A most gracious thank you to all of the families and children I have worked with over the last 16 years. You have taught me far more than I could have ever taught you.

Although not a second too early and not a moment too late, God truly does answer prayers and creates the most amazing journeys in the process. It is only through clinging to His Word and prayer that we were able to keep afloat.

For I know the plans I have for you, declares the Lord, plans to prosper you and not to harm you, plans to give you a hope and a future. Jeremiah 29:11

Appendices

Appendix 1: Schoolwork during a virus

Joshua oct 27 2010

Written Phonics

1. Write the blend your teacher says.
   Circle the special sound; mark the vowel.

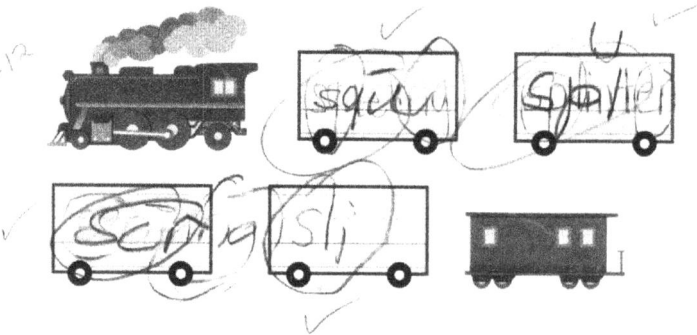

2. Write two special sounds you hear in each word your teacher says.

boing   kiking   str

ghtadu   awing   chalk

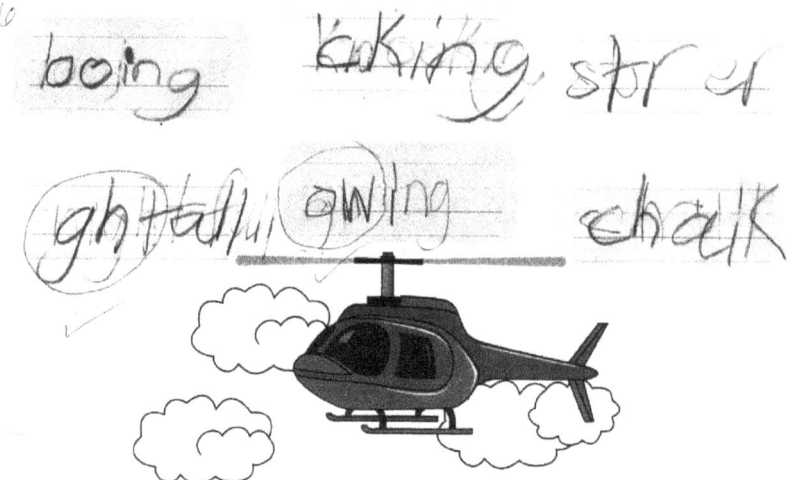

Appendix 2: Schoolwork after treatment in December